Genetic Counselling Essentials

Practice Manual for Syndromes and Inherited Disorders

Nandha Kumar S, Ph.D.
Certified Genetic Counsellor
Associate Professor, Department of Anatomy
AIIMS, Mangalagiri

&

Sangeetha A, M.D.
Certified Genetic Counsellor
Assistant Professor, Department of Anatomy
AIIMS, Mangalagiri

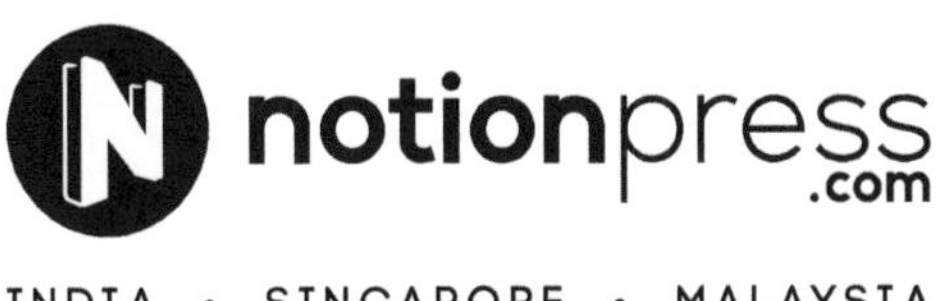

INDIA • SINGAPORE • MALAYSIA

ISBN 979-8-89984-781-3

Preface

Genetic counselling is rapidly evolving from a specialized service into an essential component of medical practice. With the increasing availability of genetic tests and the growing recognition of hereditary components in a wide range of conditions, genetic counselling plays a pivotal role in helping individuals and families understand the medical, psychological, and familial implications of genetic contributions to disease and make informed decisions.

This book, *Genetic Counselling Essentials: Practice Manual for Syndromes and Inherited Disorders,* was born out of a need we experienced in our own counselling sessions; an accessible, ready-to-use guide for those stepping into the world of genetic counselling. While existing textbooks provide extensive theoretical knowledge, the practical nuances of conducting a genetic counselling session, how to interpret results, communicate risks, support families, and plan follow-up, often remain underemphasized.

Designed for early-career genetic counsellors, postgraduate trainees, and clinicians this manual bridges the gap between theory and practice. Each chapter follows a consistent structure: Introduction, Genetic Etiology, Clinical Manifestations, and a detailed Genetic Counselling Workflow, ensuring clarity and ease of reference during counselling sessions. The disorders include autosomal, X-linked, chromosomal, developmental, reproductive, and cancer-related conditions, reflecting the diverse challenges faced in genetic counselling.

This book is not only a guide but a companion to support you during counselling sessions, while preparing for exams, and as you navigate the complexities of genetic counselling. Written by practising genetic counsellors, it offers factual knowledge, experience-based insights to help you counsel with confidence, compassion, and clarity.

We hope this manual empowers you to make informed, empathetic, and effective contributions to patient care.

– *The Authors*

Acknowledgements

We express our heartfelt gratitude to Prof. Dr. Mukesh Tripathi, former Director and CEO, AIIMS-Mangalagiri, for his foresight in recognizing the importance of genetic counselling in the genomic era. We are deeply thankful for his mentorship, which laid the foundation for the establishment of the Genetic Counselling Unit at AIIMS-Mangalagiri.

We extend our sincere gratitude to Prof. Dr. Ahanthem Santa Singh, Executive Director, AIIMS-Mangalagiri, for his continued support, guidance, and encouragement toward the growth and strengthening of genetic counselling services.

We express our profound gratitude to Dr. Joy A. Ghoshal, Dean (Research & AHS), Professor and Head, Department of Anatomy, AIIMS-Mangalagiri, for his unconditional support in obtaining administrative approvals, establishing the necessary infrastructure, and securing clearances from regulatory bodies for the successful setup of the Genetic Counselling Unit at AIIMS-Mangalagiri. Without his guidance and unwavering support, the Genetic Counselling Unit would have remained a distant dream.

We are deeply indebted to Dr. Jyoti P. Kulkarni, Professor of Anatomy and a Certified Genetic Counsellor, AIIMS-Mangalagiri, for standing with us throughout the journey of conceptualizing, establishing, and successfully running the Genetic Counselling Unit to date.

We also acknowledge with gratitude all faculty members, teaching staff, and non-teaching staff of the Department of Anatomy, AIIMS-Mangalagiri, whose cooperation and collective efforts have contributed significantly to the successful integration of genetic counselling into clinical and academic practice.

We extend our sincere thanks to the Deans, Medical Superintendents, Doctors, Nursing Officers, and the entire healthcare team at AIIMS-Mangalagiri, for their support, which has been essential for the smooth functioning of genetic counselling services.

Finally, we offer our heartfelt appreciation to the patients and their families who have attended the Genetic Counselling sessions. We are deeply grateful for their trust, openness, and willingness to engage in the counselling process. Their experiences and shared journeys continue to inspire our work and have enriched the practical insights presented in *Genetic Counselling Essentials.*

– *The Authors*

Contents

Introduction to Genetic Counselling

Scope of Genetic Counselling

- Genetic counselling is a communication process that aims to assist individuals, couples, and families in understanding the medical, psychological, and familial implications of genetic contributions to disease.
- This includes interpreting family and medical histories to assess disease risk, educating about inheritance, testing, management, and prevention options, and providing psychosocial support to facilitate informed decision-making.
- The scope of genetic counselling spans a variety of settings, including prenatal, pediatric, adult-onset, cancer genetics, infertility, and pre-symptomatic testing, and is relevant for both rare monogenic disorders and common complex diseases with genetic predispositions.

History and Evolution of the Field

- The field of genetic counselling emerged in the mid-20th century in response to advances in medical genetics and the growing need to support families with inherited conditions.
- Initially rooted in eugenics and medical genetics, the profession evolved significantly after World War II, particularly with the development of prenatal diagnostics and cytogenetics. The first

formal training programs began in the 1960s in the United States and later spread globally.

- Over time, genetic counselling has expanded from being a physician-led service to a recognized allied health profession, emphasizing non-directiveness, ethical practice, and patient-centered communication.
- Advances in genomics, such as next-generation sequencing and precision medicine, have further broadened its clinical applications and scope for its practise.

Principles of Genetic Counselling

Genetic counselling is founded on several core principles that ensure the process remains patient-centered, ethically sound, and clinically effective.

- **Non-directiveness** is a principle, where counsellors provide accurate information and emotional support but do not influence or dictate the patient's choices.
- **Respect for autonomy**, which emphasizes the individual's right to make informed decisions about their genetic health without compulsion.
- **Confidentiality** is also imperative, as sensitive genetic information must be protected and only shared with appropriate consent.
- **Informed consent**, requiring that the individual fully understand the purpose, risks, benefits, and limitations of genetic testing before proceeding.
- **Beneficence** and **non-maleficence** guide the practice—promoting the well-being of the individual while avoiding harm.
- **Cultural sensitivity, clarity in communication,** and **a commitment to ongoing education** further support responsible and effective counselling practice.

Goals and Outcomes of Genetic Counselling

- The primary goals of genetic counselling include improving understanding of genetic conditions, facilitating informed choices, promoting adaptation to the risk or presence of a disorder, and supporting autonomy.
- Outcomes may vary depending on the clinical context but often include increased genetic literacy, reduced decisional conflict, improved coping, and the formulation of proactive management or reproductive plans.
- Genetic counselling also contributes to public health through early diagnosis, cascade testing, and prevention strategies for inherited diseases, aiming to empower individuals while minimising genetic stigma or discrimination.

Role of a Genetic Counsellor

- In clinical practice, genetic counsellors function as part of a multidisciplinary healthcare team. Their roles include collecting detailed medical and family histories, constructing pedigrees, assessing recurrence risks, educating clients about genetics and available tests, obtaining informed consent, and delivering and interpreting genetic test results.
- Additionally, they provide emotional support, facilitate decision-making without compulsion, and coordinate referrals to appropriate specialists. In pediatric and adult genetics, counsellors aid in diagnosis and family screening; in prenatal settings, they support reproductive choices; and in oncology, they assess hereditary cancer risks and testing eligibility.
- Overall, they serve as key communicators between patients, families, laboratories, and clinicians.

Core Skills of a Genetic Counsellor

A genetic counsellor must possess a robust set of clinical, interpersonal, and ethical skills to navigate the complex intersection of genomics, patient care, and emotional support.

- **Communication skills** are essential, enabling the counsellor to explain complex genetic concepts in clear, accessible language while maintaining empathy and active listening.
- **Risk assessment and interpretation skills** involve collecting detailed family histories, constructing pedigrees, and applying genetic knowledge to estimate disease risks and inheritance patterns accurately.
- **Psychosocial support** is another vital competency, as genetic counsellors often help individuals cope with anxiety, grief, uncertainty, or guilt associated with a diagnosis or test result.
- **Critical thinking and decision-making skills,** especially when determining testing strategies, interpreting results, or identifying when to refer to specialists.
- **Cultural competence, ethical reasoning**, and **interdisciplinary collaboration** are increasingly important as counselling contexts become more diverse and integrated within healthcare systems.

References

1. Resta, R. G., Biesecker, B. B., Bennett, R. L., Blum, S., Hahn, S. E., Strecker, M. N., & Williams, J. L. (2006). A new definition of genetic counseling: National Society of Genetic Counselors' Task Force report. Journal of Genetic Counseling, 15(2), 77–83.
2. Middleton, A., et al. (2021). The role of genetic counsellors in genomic healthcare in the UK: A workforce survey. European Journal of Human Genetics, 29, 1261–1270.Middleton A, et al. (2020). Global

practices in genetic counseling: a systematic review. *European Journal of Human Genetics*, 28(10), 1317-1331.

3. National Society of Genetic Counselors (NSGC). (2023). *Code of Ethics.* https://www.nsgc.org/POLICY/Code-of-Ethics-Conflict-of-Interest/Code-of-Ethics
4. Biesecker, B. B., & Peters, K. F. (2001). Process studies in genetic counseling: Peering into the black box. American Journal of Medical Genetics, 106(3), 191–198.Palmer CG, et al. (2019). Facilitating informed decision-making in genomic medicine: a systematic review of the literature. *Genetics in Medicine*, 21(9), 1933-1944.
5. Skirton, H., Lewis, C., Kent, A., & Coviello, D. A. (2010). Genetic education and the challenge of genomic medicine: Development of core competences to support preparation of health professionals in Europe. European Journal of Human Genetics, 18(9), 972–977.

Genetic Counselling Workflow

Review of Medical and Family History

- Patient Information Collection: The genetic counsellor's first responsibility is to gather a thorough medical and family history from the patient, ideally covering at least three generations. This involves asking detailed questions about family member's health, consanguinity, genetic conditions, causes of death, ages of onset of diseases, and any previous genetic testing results within the family.
- Pedigree Creation: The counsellor draws a detailed pedigree chart based on the collected information, which is essential for assessing hereditary risks, inheritance patterns, and potential genetic disorders that may affect the patient or their family members.
- Risk Identification: Using this information, the counsellor identifies genetic risk factors and inheritance patterns, enabling them to make informed recommendations for diagnostic tests or preventive measures.

Discussion of Diagnosis

- Explanation of Findings: The counsellor discusses any existing or suspected diagnosis with the patient, ensuring that they understand the medical terminology, symptoms, and impact of the disorder.

- Detailed Condition Overview: They provide a comprehensive overview of the condition, including typical disease progression, severity, prognosis, and potential complications.
- Treatment and Management Options: If available, the counsellor also discusses existing treatment options, management strategies, and lifestyle adaptations that could improve the patient's quality of life.

Inheritance Pattern and Recurrence Risk Explanation

- Inheritance Mechanisms: The counsellor explains the mode of inheritance relevant to the specific condition, whether it is autosomal dominant, autosomal recessive, X-linked, mitochondrial, or multifactorial.
- Recurrence Risks: For each inheritance pattern, the counsellor discusses the likelihood of recurrence within the family, offering estimates and examples to clarify risks. For instance, in an autosomal recessive disorder, the counsellor explains the 25% recurrence risk for each child if both parents are carriers.
- Implications for Family Members: The counsellor addresses how these inheritance patterns affect extended family members, recommending testing for at-risk relatives if necessary.

Pre-Test Counselling

- Purpose of Testing: The counsellor outlines the objectives of genetic testing, such as confirming a diagnosis, identifying carrier status, or assessing risk for future offspring.
- Types of Tests: They discuss the various testing options available (e.g., diagnostic testing, carrier testing, predictive testing) and help the patient select the most appropriate one based on their goals and family history.
- Benefits, Risks, and Limitations: The counsellor explains the potential benefits of testing (e.g., informed family planning decisions, early

interventions), alongside any physical, emotional, and financial risks, as well as the limitations of certain tests.

- Informed Consent: The genetic counsellor ensures the patient's understanding of all aspects of testing and obtains informed consent, documenting the patient's choice and understanding.

Post-Test Counselling

- Review of Results: The counsellor carefully explains the test results, including positive, negative, or uncertain findings. They clarify what each result means and address any misconceptions.
- Emotional Support and Clarity: The counsellor provides emotional support as the patient processes the results, recognizing the potential psychological impact of both favourable and unfavourable findings.
- Implications for Family: They discuss how the results impact the patient's family, including whether further testing is recommended for other family members, and they review any necessary changes to risk assessment based on the results.
- Next Steps: Depending on the results, the counsellor recommends a follow-up plan that may include referrals, preventive measures, lifestyle modifications, or further monitoring.

Medical Management and Surveillance

- Coordination with Medical Professionals: The counsellor collaborates with healthcare providers, such as physicians and specialists, to review the treatment plan if the genetic test indicates a predisposition or presence of a genetic disorder.
- Surveillance Recommendations: Based on risk levels, the counsellor advises on appropriate surveillance protocols, such as regular screening tests, imaging, or laboratory tests, to monitor potential disease development.

- Preventive and Therapeutic Measures: The counsellor reviews relevant preventive options, including lifestyle changes, medication, or surgical interventions, depending on the condition and its progression.
- Compliance and Education: Counsellors stress the importance of adherence to the recommended surveillance and treatment plan, providing educational materials to help patients understand and manage their health effectively.

Reproductive and Family Planning

- Family Planning Options: The counsellor discusses reproductive options based on the genetic diagnosis and family goals. Options may include preimplantation genetic diagnosis (PGD) during in vitro fertilization (IVF), prenatal testing (such as amniocentesis or chorionic villus sampling), adoption, or using donor gametes.
- Counselling on Genetic Risks to Offspring: They explain the potential risks to offspring based on the genetic test results, empowering the patient with information on the likelihood of passing on genetic disorders.
- Assistance with Decision-Making: The counsellor supports the patient through their decision-making process, offering guidance without imposing personal biases. They address ethical considerations and respect the patient's values and beliefs.
- Referral for Further Support: If needed, the counsellor provides referrals to specialists, such as fertility experts, to support further decision-making.

Psychosocial Support

- Addressing Emotional Impact: The counsellor helps patients process the emotional effects of genetic testing, which may include anxiety, guilt, or relief. They create a safe environment for patients to express concerns and emotions.

- Family Dynamics and Communication: Counselling may extend to helping patients navigate complex family dynamics, such as how to disclose sensitive genetic information to relatives.
- Coping Strategies and Resources: The counsellor provides coping strategies to manage stress, anxiety, or other psychological challenges and directs patients to resources like support groups, therapy, or community organizations.
- Advocacy for Patient Rights: The counsellor advocates for patient rights, ensuring their access to necessary resources, understanding of privacy rights, and respect within the healthcare system.

Follow-Up and Referrals

- Scheduled Follow-Ups: The counsellor arranges follow-up appointments to reassess the patient's understanding, address any new questions, and provide continuous support.
- Coordinating with Medical Providers: They coordinate with other healthcare providers involved in the patient's care to ensure a holistic approach and relay important genetic information for integrated management.
- Specialist Referrals: Depending on the patient's needs, the counsellor may refer them to specialists, such as oncologists, neurologists, or pediatricians, based on the genetic findings and the required follow-up care.
- Long-Term Support Plan: Counsellors develop a long-term support plan, particularly for conditions that may manifest or progress over time, ensuring the patient has ongoing access to information, resources, and care as needed.

Ethical Considerations

- Informed Consent and Autonomy: The genetic counsellor ensures that patients understand the purpose, potential outcomes, and limitations of genetic testing, respecting their right to make informed decisions about their care. Non-directive counselling is a key component, where counsellors provide information and guidance without pressuring patients toward a specific decision, thereby supporting patient autonomy.

- Confidentiality and Privacy: Counsellors are responsible for maintaining strict confidentiality of patient information, particularly regarding sensitive genetic data. This includes respecting patient privacy when discussing information that could impact family members and adhering to legal privacy standards to ensure genetic data security and patient trust.

Record-Keeping

- Documentation of Counselling Sessions: The genetic counsellor meticulously records each session, including medical history, family pedigree, patient questions, consent obtained, and testing outcomes. This documentation provides a comprehensive account of the patient's genetic counselling process and serves as an important reference for continuity of care.
- Data Security and Compliance: Ensuring compliance with privacy laws, genetic counsellors maintain secure and accessible records that are only shared with authorized healthcare providers. Proper record-keeping practices help protect patient information, support accurate follow-up, and contribute to high standards of care in genetic counselling services.

References

1. Clarke, A. J. (2019). Harper's practical genetic counselling (8th ed.). CRC Press.
2. Pan, V. Y., Schuette, J. L., Wain, K. E., & Yashar, B. M. (Eds.). (2024). A guide to genetic counseling (3rd ed.). Wiley-Blackwell.

3. Hooker, G. W., Ormond, K. E., Sweet, K., & Biesecker, B. B. (2014). Teaching genomic counseling: preparing the genetic counseling workforce for the genomic era. Journal of genetic counseling, 23(4), 445–451.
4. Patch, C., & Middleton, A. (2018). Genetic counselling in the era of genomic medicine. British medical bulletin, 126(1), 27–36.
5. Hunt Brendish, K., Patel, D., Yu, K., Alexander, C. K., Lemons, J., Gunter, A., & Carmany, E. P. (2021). Genetic counseling clinical documentation: Practice Resource of the National Society of Genetic Counselors. Journal of genetic counseling, 30(5), 1336–1353.

AUTOSOMAL DOMINANT DISORDERS

List of Autosomal dominant disorders

Huntington's disease	Osteogenesis imperfecta
Marfan syndrome	Von Hippel-Lindau syndrome
Neurofibromatosis type 1	Retinoblastoma
Familial hypercholesterolemia	Noonan syndrome
Hereditary spherocytosis	Tuberous sclerosis
Polycystic kidney disease (adult onset)	Charcot-Marie-Tooth disease
Achondroplasia	Spinocerebellar ataxias (SCA)
Familial adenomatous polyposis (FAP)	Hereditary spastic paraplegia (HSP)
Ehlers-Danlos syndrome	Myotonic dystrophy
Hereditary hemorrhagic telangiectasia (HHT)	Multiple endocrine neoplasia (MEN) syndromes

General characteristics of Autosomal dominant inheritance pattern

- One mutated copy of the gene is sufficient to cause the disorder. Homozygotes for the mutant gene often die in utero or some survive with severe phenotype.

- They are often vertically transmitted (passed down from one generation to the next). Both males and females are affected equally and there is no carrier state.
- If one parent is affected (heterozygous), each child has a 50% chance of inheriting the disorder.
- Variable expressivity: the severity, age of onset, and manifestations of the disorder can vary among affected individuals, even within the same family.
- Incomplete penetrance: some individuals with the mutated gene may not express any symptoms or clinical features of the disorder.
- The disorder can arise due to a de novo mutation in the affected individual, with no family history of the condition.
- Genetic counselling is often recommended to help individuals and families understand the inheritance pattern, recurrence risks, and available options for management and prevention.

Neurofibromatosis

Introduction

- Neurofibromatosis (NF) is a group of genetic disorders characterized by the growth of tumors along nerves in the skin, brain, and other parts of the body.
- Neurofibromatosis type 1 (NF1) and Neurofibromatosis type 2 (NF2) are the two most common types, with NF1 being more prevalent.
- Both conditions show autosomal dominant inheritance with variable expressivity and high penetrance.
- Clinical features may vary widely, requiring lifelong multidisciplinary surveillance and management.

Genetic Etiology

- Neurofibromatosis type 1 (NF1) is caused by mutations in the NF1 gene, located on chromosome 17q11.2. This gene encodes for a protein called neurofibromin, which acts as a tumor suppressor and regulates cell growth and division.
- Mutations in the NF1 gene lead to a loss or dysfunction of neurofibromin, resulting in uncontrolled cell proliferation and the formation of tumors in peripheral nervous system and other tissues.

- Neurofibromatosis type 2 (NF2) is caused by mutations in the NF2 gene. The NF2 gene is located on chromosome 22q12.2 and encodes a protein called Merlin, which acts as a tumor suppressor.
- Mutations in the NF2 gene lead to the production of a non-functional or altered Merlin protein, disrupting its tumor-suppressing activity, leading to uncontrolled growth of cells, particularly Schwann cells.
- About 50% of NF1 and NF2 cases arise from spontaneous (de novo) mutations, where neither parent has the condition, but the affected individual develops it due to a new mutation in the NF1/NF2 gene.
- NF1 has a higher rate of de novo mutations (50%) than NF2 (30–50%) and mosaicism is more frequent in NF2.

Clinical manifestations of NF-1

- Café-au-lait spots (light brown skin patches)
- Neurofibromas (benign nerve tumors)
- Lisch nodules (pigmented iris hamartomas)
- Freckling in axillae or groin
- Optic pathway gliomas
- Skeletal abnormalities – scoliosis, kyphosis, sphenoid wing dysplasia
- Learning disabilities
- Macrocephaly
- Short stature
- Hypertension
- Cardiovascular abnormalities
- Increased risk of malignant peripheral nerve sheath tumors (MPNST).

Clinical manifestations of NF-2

- Bilateral Vestibular Schwannomas (Acoustic Neuromas)
- Schwannomas of cranial and spinal nerves

- Meningioma
- Ependymoma
- Cataracts, retinal abnormalities, and optic nerve meningioma
- Increased risk of malignant peripheral nerve sheath tumors.

Genetic Diagnosis

- Sequencing of the entire gene or targeted analysis for specific mutations known to be associated with NF1 and NF2. If a pathogenic variant is identified in the NF1 or NF2 gene, it confirms the diagnosis of neurofibromatosis.
- Deletion/duplication analysis for the NF1 or NF2 gene can be done using techniques such as Multiplex Ligation-dependent Probe Amplification (MLPA) or chromosomal microarray analysis (CMA).
- Mosaicism may be missed by blood testing. In such cases, tumor or affected tissue analysis may be needed for NF1 or NF2 diagnosis.

Genetic Counselling

- **Review of medical and family history**

  Detailed information about the affected individual's medical history, including symptoms (specific attention to dermatological signs, hearing loss, vestibular symptoms and tumors), age of onset, other relevant diagnostic tests or procedures performed, family history of NF1/NF2 or related conditions, using a three-generational pedigree chart and consanguinity information, should be obtained.
- **Discussion of Diagnosis**

  Explain the clinical features of NF1/NF2 and clarify any questions or uncertainties about the diagnosis. Discuss how variable expressivity and incomplete/age-dependent penetrance can affect the severity and clinical presentation of the disorder in different individuals.

- **Inheritance Pattern and Recurrence Risk**

  NF1/NF2 follows an autosomal dominant inheritance pattern, hence the individual has a 50% chance of inheriting the NF1/NF2 gene mutation from an affected parent, and 50% chance of transmitting it to each offspring. The counsellor should discuss the likelihood of other family members being affected and provide information about genetic testing options for family members who may be at risk. Explain that about 50% of NF1 and 30-50% of NF2 cases occur spontaneously (due to de novo mutation) and have no prior family history.

- **Pre-test counselling**

  Explain the role of genetic testing in confirming a diagnosis of NF1/ NF2 and determining the specific genetic mutation responsible for the condition. Discuss the benefits, limitations, and implications of genetic testing, including potential psychological and emotional considerations, and facilitate informed decision-making regarding genetic testing. Obtain informed consent before proceeding with testing.

- **Post-test counselling**

  Communicate the genetic test results to the individual or family, providing clear explanations and answering any questions or concerns that may arise. Interpret the test results in the context of the individual's medical and family history, explaining the implications of positive, negative, or inconclusive results. If pathogenic variant is found, at-risk family members should be offered genetic testing to identify those who carry the mutation and require early screening and management. Clarify that a negative genetic test result does not always rule out NF1 or NF2, especially if clinical features are present.

- **Medical Management and Surveillance**

  NF1 requires annual clinical evaluations, ophthalmologic exams, and monitoring of blood pressure, developmental milestones, and learning/developmental issues. NF2 surveillance includes annual

MRI of the brain and spine, audiology evaluations, and neurologic assessments. Early treatment of tumors, including surgical interventions, chemotherapy (e.g., selumetinib for NF1 plexiform neurofibromas), or targeted therapies (e.g., bevacizumab for NF2-related schwannomas), may be needed.

- **Reproductive and Family Planning**

  If applicable, discuss reproductive options and family planning considerations for the affected individual and other family members. Options include preimplantation genetic testing for monogenic conditions (PGT-M) with IVF, prenatal testing (CVS or amniocentesis), or the use of donor gametes. These options are especially important for individuals with severe manifestations, early-onset NF2, or those who wish to avoid passing on the condition.

- **Psychosocial Support**

  Genetic counselling should include emotional support, address body image concerns (e.g., visible neurofibromas), and provide guidance to help individuals and families cope with the challenges of living with NF1/NF2. Address any concerns, fears, or psychosocial issues that the family may be experiencing, and provide resources for additional support services, such as support groups and mental health counselling.

- **Follow-Up and Referral**

  Schedule follow-up appointments as needed to monitor the individual's condition, provide ongoing support, and address any new questions or concerns that arise. Refer them to other healthcare providers or specialists, including ophthalmologists, neurologist, dermatologist, ENT, geneticists, and mental health professionals for multidisciplinary care.

- **Documentation**

  Documentation should include a detailed family history and three-generation pedigree, along with consent forms and genetic test results. Key discussion points such as diagnosis, management plan, reproductive risks, and cascade testing recommendations must be summarized. All records should be securely stored with strict confidentiality.

References

1. Legius, E., et al. (2021). Revised diagnostic criteria for neurofibromatosis type 1 and Legius syndrome: an international consensus recommendation. Genetics in medicine : official journal of the American College of Medical Genetics, 23(8), 1506–1513.
2. Goetsch Weisman, A., Weiss McQuaid, S., Radtke, H. B., Stoll, J., Brown, B., & Gomes, A. (2023). Neurofibromatosis- and schwannomatosis-associated tumors: Approaches to genetic testing and counseling considerations. American journal of medical genetics. Part A, 191(10), 2467–2481.
3. Saleh, M., Dib, A., Beaini, S., Saad, C., Faraj, S., El Joueid, Y., Kotob, Y., Saoudi, L., & Emmanuel, N. (2023). Neurofibromatosis type 1 system-based manifestations and treatments: a review. Neurological sciences : official journal of the Italian Neurological Society and of the Italian Society of Clinical Neurophysiology, 44(6), 1931–1947.
4. Radtke, H. B., et al. (2020). Genetic Counseling for Neurofibromatosis 1, Neurofibromatosis 2, and Schwannomatosis-Practice Resource of the National Society of Genetic Counselors. Journal of genetic counseling, 29(5), 692–714.

Marfan syndrome

Introduction

- Marfan syndrome is a systemic connective tissue disorder.
- It primarily affects the skeletal, cardiovascular, and ocular systems.
- It is caused by mutations in the FBN1 gene encoding fibrillin-1.
- The condition shows variable expressivity and complete penetrance.
- Early identification is crucial to prevent life-threatening complications such as aortic dissection.

Genetic Etiology

- It is an autosomal dominant disorder.
- It is caused by mutations in the FBN1 gene, which is located on chromosome 15q21.1. The FBN1 gene encodes fibrillin-1, a glycoprotein that plays a crucial role in the formation of elastic fibers in connective tissues.
- Mutations in the FBN1 gene lead to abnormal fibrillin-1 production or function, resulting in multisystem connective tissue weakness affecting the skeletal, cardiovascular, and ocular systems.
- About 70–75% of individuals diagnosed with Marfan syndrome have an affected parent, and 25-30% are sporadic (de novo mutation).

Clinical manifestations

- Skeletal features:
    - Tall stature with long limbs (dolichostenomelia)
    - Long, thin fingers (arachnodactyly)
    - Hypermobile joints, particularly in the fingers, wrists, elbows, and knees
    - Scoliosis or abnormal curvature of the spine
    - Chest deformities, such as pectus excavatum or pectus carinatum
    - Pes planus (flat feet)
    - Positive wrist sign (Walker-Murdoch sign) and thumb sign (Steinberg sign)
- Cardiovascular features:
    - Aortic root dilation or aneurysm, which can lead to aortic dissection
    - Mitral valve prolapse
    - Aortic valve regurgitation
    - Other heart valve abnormalities
- Ocular features:
    - Ectopia lentis, or lens dislocation, which can cause blurred vision or visual disturbances
    - Myopia
    - Increased risk of retinal detachment
    - Glaucoma
    - Cataract
- Other features:
    - Dural ectasia, or enlargement of the dural sac surrounding the spinal cord, which can cause back pain or neurological symptoms

- Pulmonary abnormalities, such as spontaneous pneumothorax
- Stretch marks (striae) on the skin, especially in areas of rapid growth
- Soft, velvety skin texture
- Hernias, particularly inguinal hernias

Genetic Diagnosis

- Molecular genetic testing of FBN1 by DNA sequencing to identify point mutations and small deletions/insertions.
- Deletion/duplication analysis (e.g., MLPA or CMA) for large intragenic deletions or duplications not detected by sequencing.
- Echocardiography to assess aortic root dimensions, aortic valve morphology, and valvular involvement.
- Family screening with molecular testing is recommended if a familial variant is known.
- Ghent criteria is used for clinical diagnosis in absence of genetic confirmation.

Genetic Counselling

- **Review of medical and family history**

  Gather detailed information about the affected individual's medical history, including symptoms, age of onset, other relevant diagnostic tests or procedures performed, family history of Marfan syndrome or related conditions using a three-generational pedigree chart, and consanguinity information. Age of onset of aortic dilation/dissection, lens dislocation, retinal detachment, sudden cardiac death, and skeletal deformities in the affected family members should be noted to understand the severity and progression.

- **Discussion of Diagnosis**

  Explain what Marfan syndrome is, how it is inherited, and its associated risks, including information about the various systems that can be affected such as the cardiovascular, skeletal, ocular system, and others. How variable expressivity and incomplete penetrance can affect the severity and clinical presentation of the disorder in different individuals should be discussed.

- **Inheritance Pattern and Recurrence Risk**

  Marfan syndrome follows an autosomal dominant inheritance pattern, hence the individual has a 50% chance of inheriting the FBN1 gene mutation from an affected parent and a 50% chance of transmitting it to each offspring. The counsellor should discuss the likelihood of other family members being affected and provide information about genetic testing options for family members who may be at risk. De novo mutations may present without a family history. Hence, parental testing to determine inheritance should be considered.

- **Pre-test counselling**

  Explain the role of genetic testing in confirming a diagnosis of Marfan syndrome and determining the specific genetic mutation responsible for the condition. Discuss the benefits, limitations, and implications of genetic testing, including potential psychological and emotional considerations, and obtain informed consent to proceed with genetic testing.

- **Post-test counselling**

  Communicate the genetic test results to the individual or family, providing clear explanations and answering any questions or concerns that may arise. The counsellor helps interpret the test results in the context of the individual's medical and family history, explaining the implications of positive, negative, or inconclusive results. If pathogenic variant is found, at-risk family members should be offered genetic testing to identify those who carry the mutation and require early screening and management. For a negative result in a clinically suspected individual, the importance of regular medical check-ups should be emphasised.

- **Medical Management and Surveillance**

  Review the recommended management and surveillance protocols for individuals with Marfan syndrome and emphasize the importance of regular clinical evaluations and monitoring, such as cardiac evaluations, ophthalmologic exams, and orthopaedic assessments to manage symptoms effectively. Discuss the potential need for surgical interventions, such as aortic root replacement or lens removal, depending on the severity of the condition. Lifestyle modifications, such as avoiding strenuous physical activities and sports that may increase the risk of aortic dissection or joint injury, may be advised.

- **Reproductive and Family Planning**

  If applicable, discuss reproductive options and family planning considerations for the affected individual and other family members, including prenatal testing, preimplantation genetic diagnosis (PGD), and gamete donation or adoption. For affected women, discuss the increased maternal risk during pregnancy due to cardiovascular strain.

- **Psychosocial Support**

  Genetic counselling should include emotional support and guidance to help individuals and families cope with the challenges of living with Marfan syndrome. The counsellor should address any concerns, like body image issues, anxiety about aortic dissection, or psychosocial issues that the individuals and family may be experiencing and provide resources for additional support services, such as support groups and mental health counselling.

- **Follow-Up and Referrals**

  Schedule follow-up appointments as needed to monitor the individual's condition, provide ongoing support, and address any new questions or concerns that arise. Refer the family to specialists, including cardiologists, ophthalmologists, orthopaedic surgeons, geneticists and mental health professionals for multidisciplinary care.

- **Documentation**

  Maintain thorough documentation of the family pedigree, consent for genetic testing, test reports, discussion points, and follow-up plans. Ensure secure and confidential storage of all medical and counselling records.

References

1. Robinson, P. N., et al (2006). The molecular genetics of Marfan syndrome and related disorders. Journal of medical genetics, 43(10), 769–787.
2. Groth, K. A., et al. (2015). Prevalence, incidence, and age at diagnosis in Marfan Syndrome. Orphanet journal of rare diseases, 10, 153.
3. Marelli, S., et al. (2023). Marfan Syndrome: Enhanced Diagnostic Tools and Follow-up Management Strategies. Diagnostics (Basel, Switzerland), 13(13), 2284.
4. Monda, E., Caiazza, M., & Limongelli, G. (2024). The role of genetic testing in Marfan syndrome. Current opinion in cardiology, 39(3), 162–169.
5. von Kodolitsch, Y., et al. (2015). Perspectives on the revised Ghent criteria for the diagnosis of Marfan syndrome. The application of clinical genetics, 8, 137–155.

Achondroplasia

Introduction

- Achondroplasia is the most common form of disproportionate short stature (dwarfism).
- It is a skeletal dysplasia primarily affecting endochondral bone growth.
- Individuals present with characteristic physical features and normal intelligence.
- It is caused by mutations in the FGFR3 gene.
- Early diagnosis enables appropriate medical management and genetic counselling.

Genetic Etiology

- Achondroplasia is an autosomal dominant disorder
- It is caused by mutations in the FGFR3 gene (Fibroblast Growth Factor Receptor 3) which is located on chromosome 4p16.3. The FGFR3 gene encodes fibroblast growth factor receptor 3, which plays a crucial role in in the proliferation and differentiation of chondrocytes in the growth plates of bones.
- A single nucleotide mutation in the FGFR3 gene affects the cartilaginous ossification in developing skeleton, thereby reducing linear growth in long bones and vertebrae and premature closure of

the growth plates. However, membranous ossification in the skull and facial bones is not affected

- In about 80% of cases, the mutation is de novo in the affected individual, with no family history of the condition. In the remaining 20% of cases, the mutation is inherited from an affected parent.

Clinical manifestations

- Short stature, disproportionately short proximal limbs (rhizomelia)
- Craniofacial features: prominent forehead, midface hypoplasia, depressed nasal bridge, small upturned nose
- Skeletal manifestations: short and bowed limbs, trident hand ,short fingers and toes, enlarged joints, spinal curvature (kyphosis, lordosis, or scoliosis), limited range of motion in the joints, foramen magnum stenosis
- Neurological complications: compression of the spinal cord or nerve roots due to narrowing of the spinal canal, increased risk of hydrocephalus
- Respiratory complications: narrowing of the upper airway, leading to obstructive sleep apnea.
- Other complications: recurrent ear infections, hearing loss, obesity, delayed motor development, dental crowding, and malocclusion

Genetic Diagnosis

- Sequencing the FGFR3 gene to identify pathogenic variants (mutations) that are associated with the condition.
- Testing includes targeted analysis for specific mutations known to be associated with Achondroplasia: G1138A substitution in FGFR3 (about 98% of cases) and G1138C substitution in FGFR3 (about 1% of cases). If a pathogenic variant is identified in the FGFR3 gene, it confirms the diagnosis of Achondroplasia.

Genetic Counselling

- **Review of medical and family history**

  Gather detailed information about the affected individual's medical history, including symptoms, physical examination, other relevant diagnostic tests or procedures performed, family history of Achondroplasia or related conditions using a three-generational pedigree chart, and consanguinity information.

- **Discussion of Diagnosis**

  Explain what Achondroplasia is, how it is inherited, and its associated risks, including information about the various skeletal and non-skeletal manifestations associated with Achondroplasia, such as short stature, craniofacial features, respiratory complications, and neurological issues. Achondroplasia has high penetrance (100%) and relatively consistent and high expressivity compared to other autosomal dominant disorders.

- **Inheritance Pattern**

  Achondroplasia follows an autosomal dominant inheritance pattern, hence the individual has a 50% chance of inheriting the FGFR3 gene mutation from an affected parent and 50% chance of transmitting it to each offspring. If both parents are affected, there is a 25% chance of a child with average stature, a 50% chance of a child with Achondroplasia and a 25% chance of a child with homozygous Achondroplasia, which is lethal. The counsellor should discuss the likelihood of other family members being affected and provide information about genetic testing options for family members who may be at risk.

- **Pre-test counselling**

  Explain the role of genetic testing in confirming a diagnosis of Achondroplasia and determining the specific genetic mutation responsible for the condition. They should discuss the benefits, limitations, and implications of genetic testing, including potential psychological and emotional considerations, and obtain informed consent to proceed with genetic testing.

- **Post-test counselling**

  Communicate the genetic test results to the individual or family, providing clear explanations and answering any questions or concerns that may arise. The counsellor should help interpret the test results in the context of the individual's medical and family history, explaining the implications of positive, negative, or inconclusive results.

- **Medical Management and Surveillance**

  Review the recommended management and surveillance protocols for individuals with Achondroplasia and emphasize the importance of regular clinical evaluations and monitoring for prosthetic support, growth hormone therapy, obesity control, treatment for sleep apnea, yearly auditory evaluation and need for surgical interventions for spinal decompression or limb-lengthening procedures, depending on the severity of the condition.

- **Reproductive and Family Planning**

  If applicable, the counsellor should discuss reproductive options and family planning considerations for the affected individual and other family members, including Preimplantation Genetic Testing for Monogenic conditions (PGT-M) with IVF, prenatal diagnosis, use of donor gametes or adoption.

- **Psychosocial Support**

  Genetic counselling should include emotional support and guidance to help individuals and families cope with the challenges of living with Achondroplasia, such as body image issues, social interactions, self-esteem, and societal attitudes towards individuals with dwarfism. The counsellor should address any concerns, fears, or psychosocial issues that the family may be experiencing and provide resources for additional support services, such as support groups or mental health counselling.

- **Follow-Up and Referrals**

  Schedule follow-up appointments as needed to monitor the individual's condition, provide ongoing support, and address any new questions or concerns that arise. They may also refer the family to other healthcare providers or specialists, including orthopaedic surgeons, neurologists, ENT, pulmonologists, geneticists, and mental health professionals for multidisciplinary care.

- **Documentation**

  Document the pedigree, clinical examination findings, informed consent for testing, counselling discussions, test results, and follow-up plan. Store records securely and ensure data privacy in accordance with medical confidentiality standards.

References

1. Pauli RM. Achondroplasia: A comprehensive clinical review. Orphanet J Rare Dis. 2019;14(1):1.
2. Savarirayan, R., et al (2022). International Consensus Statement on the diagnosis, multidisciplinary management and lifelong care of individuals with achondroplasia. Nature reviews. Endocrinology, 18(3), 173–189.
3. Hoover-Fong, J., Scott, C. I., Jones, M. C., & COMMITTEE ON GENETICS (2020). Health Supervision for People With Achondroplasia. Pediatrics, 145(6), e20201010.
4. Dardenne, E., Ishiyama, N., Lin, T. A., & Lucas, M. C. (2023). Current and emerging therapies for Achondroplasia: The dawn of precision medicine. Bioorganic & medicinal chemistry, 87, 117275.

Familial Hypercholesterolemia

Introduction

- Familial Hypercholesterolemia (FH) is a common inherited disorder of lipid metabolism.
- It leads to significantly elevated levels of low-density lipoprotein cholesterol (LDL-C).
- Individuals with FH are at a markedly increased risk for premature atherosclerotic cardiovascular disease (ASCVD).
- It occurs in both heterozygous and homozygous forms, with the latter being more severe.
- Early diagnosis and intervention are critical to prevent cardiovascular complications.

Genetic Etiology

- FH is caused by mutations in the LDLR gene (85-90% of cases) on chromosome 19p13.1–13.3, which encodes the LDL receptor responsible for clearing LDL-C from the blood.
- Other mutations in the APOB (5-10% of cases) and PCSK9 (1-3% of cases) genes can also cause FH.
- Loss-of-function mutations in the LDLR or APOB genes lead to impaired clearance of LDL-C, while gain-of-function mutations in PCSK9 increase LDL-C levels.

- Individuals with homozygous FH (mutations in both alleles) experience more severe symptoms and earlier onset than heterozygous cases.

Clinical Manifestations

- Elevated LDL-C Levels: Significantly elevated LDL-C levels from birth that are resistant to diet and lifestyle changes.
- Physical Findings:

  Xanthomas: Yellowish cholesterol deposits, often found on the tendons (Achilles, hands, elbows).

  Xanthelasma: Cholesterol deposits around the eyelids.

  Corneal Arcus: A grey or white arc visible around the cornea, often observed in young adults with FH.
- Early Cardiovascular Disease (CVD): Individuals with FH are at high risk for developing coronary artery disease, myocardial infarction, and other cardiovascular complications, often before the age of 55 in men and 65 in women.
- Family History: Commonly presents with a strong family history of hypercholesterolemia or early CVD.

Genetic Diagnosis

- Blood tests showing elevated LDL-C levels (190-400 mg/dL in heterozygous FH and >500 mg/dL in homozygous FH) in individuals with a family history of CVD are used for initial diagnosis and genetic testing indications.
- Genetic testing is the gold standard for confirming a diagnosis of FH and identifying specific variants.
- Sequencing of the LDLR, APOB, and PCSK9 genes is undertaken to identify mutations.

- Deletion/duplication analysis of LDLR by the MLPA method may be conducted if sequencing is inconclusive.
- Cascade screening of first-degree relatives is strongly recommended if a pathogenic variant is identified, as early intervention can significantly reduce CVD risk.

Genetic Counselling

- **Review of Medical and Family History**

  A detailed three-generation pedigree should be constructed to identify affected and at-risk individuals. Document any history of premature cardiovascular events, unexplained sudden cardiac death, severe hypercholesterolemia, or characteristic physical signs (e.g., xanthomas). Information on consanguinity and lipid-lowering treatment history should be recorded.

- **Discussion of Diagnosis**

  Explain the genetic basis of FH, its autosomal dominant inheritance pattern, and how it impacts cholesterol metabolism. Provide an overview of clinical manifestations and discuss both heterozygous and homozygous FH. Explain that FH can be suspected and diagnosed clinically based on elevated LDL-C, family history, and physical signs, and that these criteria guide further evaluation and treatment.

- **Inheritance Pattern and Recurrence Risk**

  Since FH is autosomal dominant, each child of an affected individual has a 50% chance of inheriting the mutation and 50% chance of transmitting it to each offspring. Emphasize that those with homozygous FH (two mutations) will have more severe symptoms and risks. The variability in expression should also be discussed.

- **Pre-test Counselling**

  Discuss the purpose of genetic testing, its potential outcomes, limitations, and implications. Obtain informed consent for genetic testing and address the emotional and psychological impact of an FH diagnosis, especially regarding early onset CVD risks.

- **Post-test Counselling**

  Communicate the genetic test results, clarifying positive, negative, or inconclusive findings and their relevance to cardiovascular risk. If a mutation is identified, recommend cascade testing for at-risk relatives and provide information on preventative care to reduce the risk of CVD. Emphasize the importance of identifying heterozygous individuals early for timely intervention and significant reduction in their CVD risk. For a negative result in a clinically suspected individual, the importance of regular medical check-ups should be outlined.

- **Medical Management and Surveillance**

  Emphasize the importance of lifestyle modifications (diet, exercise, smoking cessation), early management and routine surveillance. Treatment often includes statins or other lipid-lowering therapies. Provide recommendations for routine blood lipid profile and cardiac monitoring. Emphasize the lifelong nature of treatment and the importance of adherence.

- **Reproductive and Family Planning**

  If applicable, discuss options for family planning, such as preimplantation genetic diagnosis (PGD) or prenatal testing to avoid transmission of FH to offspring, especially if both parents are affected.

- **Psychosocial Support**

  Provide support for families coping with the risks of CVD and discuss any anxieties related to lifestyle adjustments, especially in young individuals diagnosed with FH. Recommend support groups, mental health resources, and educational programs to help individuals and families manage the condition effectively.

- **Follow-Up and Referrals**

  Schedule follow-up sessions as needed to monitor adherence to treatment plans and lipid-lowering therapies. Refer patients to specialists, such as dietitian, endocrinologist and cardiologists for comprehensive care and personalised management.

- **Documentation**

  Accurate documentation of family history, clinical findings, genetic test results, and informed consent is important. Maintain updated surveillance and treatment records. All information must be stored securely with strict confidentiality.

References

1. Goldberg, A. C., et al & National Lipid Association Expert Panel on Familial Hypercholesterolemia (2011). Familial hypercholesterolemia: screening, diagnosis and management of pediatric and adult patients: clinical guidance from the National Lipid Association Expert Panel on Familial Hypercholesterolemia. Journal of clinical lipidology, 5(3 Suppl), S1–S8.
2. Watts, G. F., et al. (2023). International Atherosclerosis Society guidance for implementing best practice in the care of familial hypercholesterolaemia. Nature reviews. Cardiology, 20(12), 845–869.
3. Tada, H., Kawashiri, M. A., Nohara, A., Sekiya, T., Watanabe, A., & Takamura, M. (2024). Genetic Counseling and Genetic Testing for Familial Hypercholesterolemia. Genes, 15(3), 297.
4. Sturm, A.C. The Role of Genetic Counselors for Patients with Familial Hypercholesterolemia. Curr Genet Med Rep 2, 68–74 (2014).

Huntington Disease

Introduction

- Huntington disease (HD) is a progressive neurodegenerative disorder characterized by motor dysfunction, cognitive decline, and psychiatric disturbances.
- It typically presents in mid-adulthood but may also appear in juvenile or late-onset forms.
- HD is inherited in an autosomal dominant pattern and has a significant psychosocial impact on affected individuals and families.

Genetic Etiology

- Caused by a CAG trinucleotide repeat expansion in the HTT gene located on chromosome 4p16.3.
- Normal alleles contain <26 CAG repeats; disease-causing alleles have ≥36 repeats.
- Intermediate alleles (27–35) do not cause disease but are unstable and may expand into the disease-causing range in future generations
- Larger repeat sizes are associated with earlier onset and faster progression of the disease due to genetic anticipation.

Clinical Manifestation

- Motor symptoms: chorea, dystonia, bradykinesia, dysphagia and impaired voluntary movements.
- Cognitive features: executive dysfunction, memory impairment, and eventual dementia.
- Psychiatric symptoms: depression, irritability, anxiety, obsessive-compulsive traits, apathy and psychosis.
- Juvenile HD: rigidity, seizures, and cognitive decline presenting before age 20.

Genetic Diagnosis

- Molecular genetic testing of the HTT gene is the definitive test, using PCR and fragment analysis to assess CAG repeat number.
- Predictive testing is available for at-risk asymptomatic individuals with a family history of HD.
- Prenatal testing and preimplantation genetic testing (PGT) can be considered for family planning.

Genetic Counselling

- **Review of Medical and Family History**

  A three-generation pedigree should be constructed to document the inheritance pattern and age of onset in affected individuals. Consanguinity, age of death, psychiatric illness, suicide attempts, and other neurodegenerative symptoms should be recorded. Confirming a clinical diagnosis in the family strengthens the basis for genetic testing and counselling.

- **Discussion of Diagnosis**

  Explain the genetic basis of HD, emphasizing the pathogenic CAG repeat expansion in the HTT gene. The diagnosis is linked to the presence of ≥36 repeats. Symptoms and typical age of onset correlate with repeat length and family history, supporting the clinical and molecular diagnosis. Explain that the test identifies the presence of the mutation, but does not predict the exact age of onset or specific symptom progression, especially for repeat sizes between 36-50.

- **Inheritance Pattern and Recurrence Risk**

  HD follows an autosomal dominant inheritance pattern, where each child of an affected individual has a 50% chance of inheriting the mutant allele. Genetic anticipation is noted, particularly in paternal transmission, with earlier onset and/or more severe symptoms in successive generations due to expansion of the CAG repeat during spermatogenesis.

- **Pre-test Counselling**

  Counselling prior to testing must facilitate informed decision making and address the profound psychological implications of learning one's genetic status. For predictive testing in asymptomatic individuals, a multi-step process involving neurological evaluation, psychological/psychiatric evaluation, and multiple counselling sessions is mandatory to ensure the individual is making an informed and considered decision. Predictive testing is not recommended for minors.

- **Post-test Counselling**

  Results should be communicated with sensitivity and ample support. A positive result confirms future disease development, though age of onset is variable. Negative results relieve transmission risk. Intermediate alleles (27–35 CAG repeats) pose uncertain implications and need careful explanation regarding their stability and potential for expansion in offspring. Refer to guidelines for intermediate allele counselling. Cascade testing should be discussed for at-risk relatives.

- **Medical Management and Surveillance**

  There is currently no cure, but symptomatic treatment can significantly improve quality of life. Neurology follow-up is essential for motor symptoms, and new therapies targeting chorea are available (e.g., tetrabenazine, deutetrabenazine, valbenazine). Psychiatric care is vital for managing mood and behavioural changes. Speech, physical, and occupational therapy are often beneficial for maintaining function. Nutritional support is needed due to weight loss and dysphagia.

- **Reproductive and Family Planning**

  Counsellors should discuss reproductive options, including preimplantation genetic diagnosis (PGD) and prenatal testing for individuals at risk of transmitting HD. Individuals should be supported in considering options like gamete donation and adoption.

- **Psychosocial Support**

  Living with or at risk for HD can cause significant psychological distress, including depression, anxiety, and anticipatory grief. Referral to support groups, and mental health professionals should be made. Family counselling can address relationship stress and caregiving burden.

- **Follow-Up and Referrals**

  Regular follow-up should involve neurology, psychiatry, genetics, social work, nutritionists, and palliative care specialists (as the disease progresses). Genetic counselling should be revisited at reproductive decision points, disease progression stages, or as new treatments/ research emerges.

- **Documentation**

  Thorough documentation must include the pedigree, informed consent for testing, test reports, counselling notes summarizing key discussions, and a structured follow-up plan. All records should be securely stored with confidentiality.

References

1. Ross, C. A., et al. (2014). Huntington disease: natural history, biomarkers and prospects for therapeutics. Nature reviews. Neurology, 10(4), 204–216.
2. Bachoud-Lévi, A. C., et al (2019). International Guidelines for the Treatment of Huntington's Disease. Frontiers in neurology, 10, 710.
3. Migliore, S., Jankovic, J., & Squitieri, F. (2019). Genetic Counseling in Huntington's Disease: Potential New Challenges on Horizon?. Frontiers in neurology, 10, 453.
4. Semaka, A., & Hayden, M. R. (2014). Evidence-based genetic counselling implications for Huntington disease intermediate allele predictive test results. Clinical genetics, 85(4), 303–311.

AUTOSOMAL RECESSIVE DISORDERS

List of Autosomal recessive disorders

Cystic Fibrosis	Galactosemia
Sickle Cell Anemia	Ataxia-Telangiectasia
Tay-Sachs Disease	Fanconi Anemia
Phenylketonuria (PKU)	Mucopolysaccharidoses
Thalassemia	Glycogen Storage Disease Type I
Albinism	Maple Syrup Urine Disease (MSUD)
Gaucher Disease	Hereditary Fructose Intolerance
Wilson Disease	Homocystinuria
Spinal Muscular Atrophy (SMA)	Congenital Adrenal Hyperplasia (CAH)

General characteristics of Autosomal recessive inheritance pattern

- An individual must inherit two mutated copies of the gene, one from each parent, to develop the disorder. Individuals with one normal copy and one mutated copy are carriers and typically do not exhibit symptoms.

- If both parents are carriers of the mutated gene, each pregnancy has a 25% risk of having an affected child, a 50% chance of having an unaffected carrier child, and a 25% chance of having an unaffected noncarrier child. If one parent is a carrier and the other is affected, then the risk of having an affected child is 50%.
- Consanguineous parents have a higher risk of having children with autosomal recessive disorders. Affected individuals typically have unaffected parents who are carriers of the mutated gene.
- It is not typically characterized by vertical transmission, it often appears to "skip" generations. Affected individuals usually have unaffected parents.
- Both males and females are affected equally.
- Variable expressivity: the severity, age of onset, and manifestations of the disorder can vary among affected individuals, even within the same family.
- Penetrance is usually complete, but subtle or subclinical manifestations may lead to underdiagnosis in some carriers or mildly affected individuals.
- Genetic counselling is often recommended to help individuals and families understand the inheritance pattern, recurrence risks, and available options for management and prevention.

Cystic Fibrosis

Introduction

- Cystic Fibrosis (CF) is a common autosomal recessive genetic disorder affecting the respiratory, gastrointestinal, and reproductive systems.
- It is caused by mutations in the CFTR gene, located on chromosome 7q31, leading to defective chloride transport across epithelial cells.
- The disease primarily affects populations of European descent but can be seen globally.
- Early diagnosis and multidisciplinary care are critical for improved outcomes significantly increased life expectancy.

Genetic Etiology

- The CFTR gene encodes the cystic fibrosis transmembrane conductance regulator protein, which regulates the movement of salt and water in and out of cells.
- The most common mutation is ΔF508, which leads to malfunctioning of chloride channels, resulting in thick and sticky mucus buildup in various organs.
- Other common mutations include G542X, G551D, and N1303K
- More than 2000 CFTR mutations have been identified, though not all are disease-causing. Class I to Class VI mutation categories define severity based on protein function.

- CF affects multiple organs due to impaired mucus clearance, leading to recurrent infections, malabsorption, and inflammation, with serious implications for the lungs and pancreas.

Clinical Manifestations

- Respiratory Symptoms:
    - Persistent cough producing thick mucus.
    - Frequent lung infections, including pneumonia and bronchitis.
    - Shortness of breath and wheezing.
    - Nasal polyps and chronic sinusitis
- Digestive Symptoms:
    - Difficulty in digesting food, leading to malnutrition and poor growth.
    - Pancreatic insufficiency and fat-soluble vitamin deficiencies (A, D, E, and K).
    - Greasy and bulky stools.
    - Liver disease (ranging from fatty liver to cirrhosis).
- Other Features:
    - Salty-tasting skin due to increased salt content in sweat.
    - Male infertility due to congenital absence of the vas deferens (CBAVD).
    - Female subfertility (due to thick cervical mucus).
    - CF-related diabetes (CFRD)
    - Osteopenia and osteoporosis in adults.
    - Digital clubbing
    - Meconium ileus in neonates

Genetic Diagnosis

- Genetic Testing for CFTR Mutations:
  - CFTR gene sequencing, multiplex mutation panels, deletion/duplication analysis are used to identify specific mutations associated with CF.
  - Carrier screening for family members is offered to identify asymptomatic carriers.
- Sweat Test: Sweat chloride level >60 mmol/L is diagnostic of CF in symptomatic individuals.
- Newborn Screening: The initial step measures IRT (Immunoreactive Trypsinogen test), a protein produced by the pancreas that is often elevated in babies with CF. If IRT levels are elevated, a genetic test is done to identify CFTR mutations.

Genetic Counselling

- **Review of Medical and Family History**

  Comprehensive review should include a three-generation pedigree to assess for consanguinity and any history of unexplained infant deaths, unexplained bronchiectasis, chronic pancreatitis, gastrointestinal issues and fertility status should be recorded. Carrier status and ethnic background should be documented.

- **Discussion of Diagnosis**

  Counsellors should explain that CF is a multisystem disorder primarily affecting the lungs and pancreas, caused by defective CFTR protein. Diagnosis is based on clinical features, sweat chloride testing, and confirmation via genetic testing. Emphasize the role of specific CFTR mutations in disease severity, and how genotype often correlates with phenotype, particularly for pancreatic status and responsiveness to CFTR modulator therapies.

- **Inheritance Pattern and Recurrence Risk**

  As an autosomal recessive disorder, CF requires mutations in both copies of the CFTR gene for the disease to manifest. Each child of carrier parents has a 25% chance of having CF (affected), a 50% chance of being a carrier, and a 25% chance of being unaffected. Genetic counselling should include discussion on population-specific carrier frequencies and recurrence risks in future pregnancies.

- **Pre-test Counselling**

  Pre-test discussions must include the purpose of testing (e.g., diagnostic testing , carrier screening, prenatal diagnosis), possible outcomes (positive, negative, VUS), and limitations. Informed consent should be obtained prior to genetic testing. Discuss implications for family members and options based on potential results.

- **Post-test Counselling**

  Results should be clearly communicated. If a pathogenic CFTR mutation is identified, recommend cascade carrier testing for siblings and extended family. In cases of VUS (variant of uncertain significance), explain limitations and the need for functional or segregation studies, emphasizing that VUS results generally do not change clinical management unless reclassified. Address psychosocial implications for diagnosed individuals and family.

- **Medical Management and Surveillance**

  Highlight the importance of comprehensive care, including respiratory therapies, enzyme supplements, CFTR modulators and infection prevention. Recommend regular monitoring and multidisciplinary care with pulmonologists, gastroenterologists, dietitians, and other specialists for multidisciplinary management.

- **Reproductive and Family Planning**

  Discuss options such as preimplantation genetic diagnosis (PGD) and prenatal genetic testing to help prevent transmission of CF to offspring. For couples at risk, in vitro fertilization (IVF) combined with PGD can be used to select embryos without CFTR mutations. In affected males with CBAVD, reproductive options include surgical sperm retrieval techniques followed by assisted reproduction. In affected females, techniques to bypass thick cervical mucus, such as intrauterine insemination (IUI) or IVF, may be considered to achieve biological parenthood. Donor gametes or adoption are alternatives for couples with high recurrence risk

- **Psychosocial Support**

  Psychological support should be offered to patients and families to address chronic illness burden, treatment fatigue, and guilt or anxiety. Refer them to CF-specific support networks and family counselling. School and vocational counselling may also be needed as the child grows to ensure appropriate accommodations and opportunities.

- **Follow-Up and Referrals**

  Regular follow-up should include pediatrician, clinical geneticist, pulmonologist, gastroenterologist, dietitian, endocrinologist, social worker, and other specialists as needed, for comprehensive management. Family members found to be carriers should be referred for genetic counselling and reproductive planning.

- **Documentation**

  Document all genetic counselling sessions, including the pedigree, risk assessment, testing details, consent forms, and discussion summaries. Genetic test reports should be securely stored, and cascade testing plans noted for future reference.

References

1. Grasemann, H., & Ratjen, F. (2023). Cystic Fibrosis. The New England journal of medicine, 389(18), 1693–1707.
2. Farrell PM, et al. (2017). Diagnosis of Cystic Fibrosis: Consensus Guidelines from the Cystic Fibrosis Foundation. *J Pediatr*. 181S:S4–S15.e1.
3. Bieth, E., Nectoux, J., Girardet, A., Gruchy, N., Mittre, H., Laurans, M., Guenet, D., Brouard, J., & Gerard, M. (2020). Genetic counseling for cystic fibrosis: A basic model with new challenges. Archives de pediatrie : organe officiel de la Societe francaise de pediatrie, 27 Suppl 1, eS30–eS34.
4. McGlynn, J., DeCelie-Germana, J. K., Kier, C., & Langfelder-Schwind, E. (2023). Reproductive Counseling and Care in Cystic Fibrosis: A Multidisciplinary Approach for a New Therapeutic Era. Life (Basel, Switzerland), 13(7), 1545.

Sickle Cell Anemia

Introduction

- Sickle Cell Anemia (SCA) is a hereditary hemoglobinopathy characterized by chronic hemolytic anemia, episodic pain crises, and multi-organ complications.
- It predominantly affects individuals of African, Mediterranean, Middle Eastern, and Indian descent.
- The condition arises due to a structural variant in the beta-globin chain of hemoglobin.

Genetic Etiology

- Sickle Cell Anemia (SCA) is an autosomal recessive disorder caused by mutations in the HBB gene on chromosome 11p15.5, leading to the production of an abnormal hemoglobin known as hemoglobin S (HbS).
- The most common mutation in SCA is a single nucleotide substitution (GAG to GTG) in the HBB gene at codon 6 of the β-globin chain, resulting in the substitution of glutamic acid by valine in the β-globin protein. This leads to the production of HbS instead of normal hemoglobin A.
- Under low oxygen conditions, HbS molecules polymerize (stick together) forming rigid fibers, causing red blood cells to become rigid

and crescent or "sickle" shaped. These misshapen cells are less flexible and can block blood flow in small capillaries, leading to pain and damage in various organs.

- In homozygous individuals (HbSS genotype), SCA manifests clinically. Compound heterozygotes (e.g., HbSC disease, HbS/β-thalassemia) may have milder phenotypes but are still considered forms of sickle cell disease (SCD).
- Sickle cell trait (HbAS) is a carrier state, where individuals are usually asymptomatic but can pass the HbS mutation to their children.

Clinical Manifestations

- Vaso-occlusive crises (VOCs): Episodes of severe pain in bones, chest, and abdomen due to blockages in blood vessels.
- Chronic anemia: Resulting from the rapid breakdown (hemolysis) of sickled red blood cells, leading to a shortened red blood cell lifespan.
- Jaundice and yellowing of the eyes due to hemolysis.
- Delayed growth and puberty in children.
- Increased infection risk due to functional asplenia (loss of spleen function).
- Acute chest syndrome: Chest pain, fever, and difficulty breathing, which can be life-threatening.
- Organ damage: Long-term damage to the spleen (autosplenectomy), lung, liver, kidneys, and other organs.
- Stroke risk: Due to blood vessel occlusions in the brain, including both ischemic and hemorrhagic strokes.
- Priapism
- Leg ulcers
- Gallstones
- Avascular necrosis of femoral head and retinopathy

Genetic Diagnosis

- Hemoglobin electrophoresis or high-performance liquid chromatography (HPLC) to identify the presence of HbS and differentiate it from other hemoglobins (e.g., HbA, HbF, HbC, HbE).
- Targeted HBB gene sequencing and deletion/duplication analysis by the MLPA method to confirm the presence of the sickle cell mutation.
- Newborn screening: Routine testing for sickle cell anemia (hemoglobin electrophoresis) enables early detection and management.

Genetic Counselling

- **Review of Medical and Family History**

  The counselling process should begin with a comprehensive review of the proband's medical history and a detailed three-generation pedigree. Information on consanguinity, previous history of anemia, unexplained jaundice, pain crises, transfusions, splenectomy, chronic organ damage, or family members with known hemoglobinopathies should be recorded.

- **Discussion of Diagnosis**

  Explain the genetic basis of SCA, its autosomal recessive inheritance, and how HbS affects blood cells. Clarify that both parents must carry one copy of the mutation (sickle cell trait) for the child to have SCA. Emphasize that individuals with sickle cell trait (heterozygotes) are usually asymptomatic but may have complications under extreme conditions (e.g., high altitude, dehydration, intense exertion).

- **Inheritance Pattern and Recurrence Risk**

  Sickle Cell Anemia follows an autosomal recessive inheritance pattern. If both parents are carriers (HbAS), each child in every pregnancy has a 25% chance of being affected (HbSS), a 50% chance of being a carrier (HbAS), and a 25% chance of being unaffected (HbAA). In cases of compound heterozygosity (e.g., one parent with HbAS and another with HbAC or beta-thalassemia trait), other clinically significant genotypes like HbSC disease or HbS/β-thalassemia may arise, with varying severity but still classified as sickle cell disease.

- **Pre-test Counselling**

  Counselling should cover the implications of carrier or disease status for the individual being tested, the potential outcomes of testing (e.g., positive, negative, carrier, VUS), psychological impact (e.g., anxiety, guilt, relief), and relevance for reproductive planning. Carrier screening is strongly recommended for individuals of high-prevalence ethnic backgrounds. Before genetic testing, informed consent must be obtained.

- **Post-test Counselling**

  Once results are available, clear communication regarding the individual's status is essential. For those identified as carriers or affected, cascade testing for siblings and other at-risk family members is recommended. Counsellors should provide information about implications for management options, including specific risks associated with different genotypes (e.g., HbSS vs. HbSC) and family planning.

- **Medical Management and Surveillance**

  Emphasize comprehensive care including regular health check-ups, hydration, infection prevention (vaccinations, prophylactic antibiotics), and pain management. Review treatment options such as hydroxyurea, blood transfusions, and, in some cases, bone marrow or stem cell transplantation. Provide guidance on recognizing signs of complications, such as acute chest syndrome or severe pain crises, which may require immediate medical attention.

- **Reproductive and Family Planning**

  Discuss family planning options, including preimplantation genetic diagnosis (PGD) for those wishing to avoid passing on SCA to their offspring. Explain prenatal diagnosis options such as chorionic villus sampling (CVS) and amniocentesis to determine fetal status. Outline alternatives such as gamete donation or adoption for couples who wish to avoid transmitting the genetic condition.

- **Psychosocial Support**

  Living with a chronic, painful, and potentially life-threatening illness has significant emotional and social impacts. Genetic counsellors should connect patients and families with local support groups, and mental health services. Educational support for affected children, vocational counselling, and support for caregivers can reduce stigma and improve quality of life.

- **Follow-Up and Referrals**

  Schedule regular follow-up appointments to monitor the individual's condition, offer ongoing support, and provide access to resources and information. Refer to specialists such as hematologists, pulmonologists, ophthalmologists, nephrologists, neurologists, cardiologists for multidisciplinary care.

- **Documentation**

  Accurate documentation of the family pedigree, clinical findings, counselling discussions, test consent, and results is critical. Records should include the management plan and follow-up strategy and must be securely stored while maintaining confidentiality.

References

1. Ware, R. E., de Montalembert, M., Tshilolo, L., & Abboud, M. R. (2017). Sickle cell disease. Lancet (London, England), 390(10091), 311–323.
2. National Institutes of Health. Evidence-Based Management of Sickle Cell Disease: Expert Panel Report, 2014.
3. Sickle cell disease. (2018). Nature reviews. Disease primers, 4, 18011.

4. Brandow, A. M., & Liem, R. I. (2022). Advances in the diagnosis and treatment of sickle cell disease. Journal of hematology & oncology, 15(1), 20.

5. Aggarwal, P., & Bhat, D. (2023). Genetic counseling in sickle cell disease: Insights from the Indian tribal population. Journal of community genetics, 14(4), 345–353.

Thalassemia

Introduction

- Thalassemia is a group of inherited blood disorders characterized by defective synthesis of one or more globin chains of hemoglobin.
- It results in chronic anemia due to ineffective erythropoiesis and hemolysis.
- The condition is highly prevalent in the Mediterranean, Middle Eastern, South Asian, and Southeast Asian populations.
- Two major types are recognized based on the affected globin chain: α-thalassemia and β-thalassemia.

Genetic Etiology

- Thalassemia is an autosomal recessive blood disorder caused by mutations affecting the production of hemoglobin, the oxygen-carrying protein in red blood cells.
- Thalassemia results from mutations in the genes that code for either the alpha (α) or beta (β) globin chains of hemoglobin.
- Mutations in these genes lead to alpha-thalassemia (mutations in the HBA1 and HBA2 genes on chromosome 16) or beta-thalassemia (mutations in the HBB gene on chromosome 11).
- Thalassemia minor (heterozygous) is characterized by the inheritance of one mutated beta-globin gene, typically resulting in mild or no

symptoms and requiring little to no treatment. It is often diagnosed through routine blood tests showing microcytic hypochromic anemia and elevated hemoglobin A2 (HbA2) levels.

- Thalassemia major (homozygous) involves inheriting two mutated beta-globin genes, leading to severe anemia that manifests in early childhood, requiring regular lifelong blood transfusions and intensive medical management. Patients with thalassemia major experience significant complications, including growth delays and organ damage due to iron overload from transfusions.
- Alpha-thalassemia severity ranges from asymptomatic silent carriers (one affected gene) to mild alpha-thalassemia trait (two affected genes), moderate to severe HbH disease (three affected genes), and lethal hydrops fetalis (four affected genes).
- Reduced or absent production of one or more globin chains leads to an imbalance in globin chain synthesis. This results in the precipitation of the unpaired, excess globin chains within red blood cell precursors, causing ineffective erythropoiesis and increased red blood cell fragility and premature destruction (hemolysis). This ultimately leads to anemia.

Clinical Manifestations

- Mild to severe Anemia: Symptoms range from mild microcytic anemia in thalassemia minor/trait to severe, transfusion-dependent anemia in beta-thalassemia major and HbH disease.
- Fatigue and weakness: Due to chronic anemia, patients may experience tiredness, reduced stamina, and exercise intolerance.
- Jaundice and pallor: Resulting from rapid breakdown of red blood cells and ineffective erythropoiesis.
- Bone deformities: Enlarged or distorted facial and cranial bones ("chipmunk facies"), thinning of cortical bone, and susceptibility to fractures due to compensatory bone marrow expansion.

- Growth delays: Particularly in children with more severe forms, such as beta-thalassemia major, often compounded by iron overload and endocrine dysfunction.
- Splenomegaly and hepatomegaly: Enlargement of the spleen and liver due to increased destruction of red blood cells and extramedullary hematopoiesis.
- Iron overload (hemosiderosis): Due to frequent blood transfusions, which can lead to complications in the heart, liver, and endocrine system.
- Gallstones: Increased risk due to chronic hemolysis and elevated bilirubin levels.
- Infections: Increased susceptibility, particularly in splenectomized patients.

Genetic Diagnosis

- Complete blood count (CBC) and red blood cell Indices: Often the first indicator, showing microcytic (low MCV) and hypochromic (low MCH) red blood cells, even in carriers.
- Hemoglobin electrophoresis or HPLC: Identifies abnormal hemoglobin types and quantifies HbA, HbF, and HbA2.
- DNA sequencing analysis of HBA1, HBA2, and HBB genes: Used to identify specific deletions or point mutations associated with alpha- or beta-thalassemia, which is crucial for definitive diagnosis and carrier identification.
- For alpha-thalassemia, deletional mutations are common and can be identified by gap-PCR or MLPA.
- Prenatal diagnosis: Chorionic villus sampling (CVS) or amniocentesis can detect mutations in the fetus if both parents are carriers.
- Carrier screening: Genetic testing to identify asymptomatic carriers, especially in high-risk populations, is vital for genetic counselling and family planning.

Genetic Counselling

- **Review of Medical and Family History**

  Obtain a detailed family history to assess patterns of thalassemia or related hematological conditions. A three-generation pedigree, along with consanguinity information, should be drawn to identify family members who may be carriers or affected. Details of unexplained anemia, jaundice, splenectomy, history of hydrops fetalis, and stillbirth must be noted.

- **Discussion of Diagnosis**

  Explain the genetic basis of thalassemia, its autosomal recessive inheritance, and how mutations disrupt hemoglobin production. Provide an overview of the clinical spectrum from thalassemia minor/trait to beta-thalassemia major and alpha-thalassemia (including HbH disease and hydrops fetalis).

- **Inheritance Pattern and Recurrence Risk**

  Emphasize on autosomal recessive inheritance: if both parents are carriers, each child has a 25% chance of having a severe form of thalassemia (affected), a 50% chance of being a carrier, and a 25% chance of being unaffected (non-carrier).

- **Pre-test Counselling**

  Informed consent must be obtained before genetic testing. The session should discuss the purpose of testing, implications for personal health (if a carrier or affected), implications for family planning, and potential emotional impact.

- **Post-test Counselling**

  Results should be clearly communicated, including carrier, affected, or normal status. For affected individuals or identified carriers, cascade testing should be offered to at-risk relatives. If both partners are carriers, reproductive options should be explored in detail, ensuring understanding of all choices. Support should be provided to process the implications of the results, addressing potential anxiety or guilt.

- **Medical Management and Surveillance**

  Review treatment options such as regular blood transfusions, iron chelation therapy to manage iron overload, and potential bone marrow or stem cell transplantation for severe cases. Emphasize the importance of regular monitoring and multidisciplinary care involving hematologists, hepatologists, nutritionists, and endocrinologists.

- **Reproductive and Family Planning**

  Discuss reproductive options, including preimplantation genetic diagnosis (PGD) for those wanting to avoid passing on thalassemia to their children. Cover prenatal testing options like chorionic villus sampling (CVS) and amniocentesis to detect the condition in utero. Outline alternatives such as gamete donation or adoption.

- **Psychosocial Support**

  Living with or raising a child with a chronic, lifelong, and often demanding condition such as thalassemia can be emotionally, financially, and socially taxing. Genetic counsellors should connect patients and families with local and national support groups and community networks to provide emotional support, shared experiences, and practical advice. Counselling should address anxiety, grief, guilt, or stigma and offer referrals to mental health professionals if needed.

- **Follow-Up and Referrals**

  Schedule regular follow-up appointments to assess ongoing needs, monitor treatment adherence, and address new concerns. Refer to specialists, including hematologists, hepatologists, cardiologists, endocrinologists, and support services, for coordinated care.

- **Documentation**

  Counselling sessions should be meticulously documented, including family history, clinical findings, consent for testing, discussion points, test results, and follow-up plan. Records must be stored securely with confidentiality.

References

1. Kattamis, A., Kwiatkowski, J. L., & Aydinok, Y. (2022). Thalassaemia. The lancet, 399(10343), 2310-2324.
2. Taher, A. T., Musallam, K. M., & Cappellini, M. D. (2021). β-Thalassemias. The New England journal of medicine, 384(8), 727–743.
3. Farmakis, D., et al. (2022). 2021 Thalassaemia International Federation Guidelines for the Management of Transfusion-dependent Thalassemia. HemaSphere, 6(8), e732.
4. Cao A. (2002). Carrier screening and genetic counselling in beta-thalassemia. International journal of hematology, 76 Suppl 2, 105–113.

Spinal Muscular Atrophy

Introduction

- Spinal Muscular Atrophy (SMA) is a group of inherited neurodegenerative disorders characterized by progressive muscle weakness due to degeneration of lower alpha motor neurons.
- It primarily affects infants and children but has variable age of onset and severity depending on the subtype.
- SMA is one of the most common fatal autosomal recessive conditions in infancy.
- Advances in molecular diagnostics and therapy have significantly improved outcomes for affected individuals.

Genetic Etiology

- SMA is primarily caused by biallelic mutations (most commonly homozygous deletions) in the SMN1 gene located on chromosome 5q13.
- This gene encodes the survival motor neuron (SMN) protein, which is critical for the maintenance of motor neurons. Loss of function in both SMN1 alleles leads to a deficiency of SMN protein, causing motor neuron degeneration.
- The SMN2 gene produces limited full-length SMN protein due to alternative splicing, but can partially compensate for SMN1 loss.

- The number of SMN2 gene copies (typically 1 to 4 or more) impacts disease severity, with more copies generally resulting in a milder phenotype due to increased production of functional SMN protein.

Clinical Manifestations

- Muscle Weakness and Atrophy: Weakness typically starts proximally (shoulders, hips) and progresses over time, leading to difficulties with movement and posture, and in severe cases, loss of motor milestones.
- Types of SMA:
  - Type 0 (Prenatal Onset): Very severe, rare form with onset in utero or at birth. Severe weakness, arthrogryposis (joint contractures), and often lethal within weeks to months due to respiratory failure.
  - Type 1 (Infantile-Onset): Severe form presenting within the first 6 months, with significant muscle weakness and respiratory difficulties.
  - Type 2 (Intermediate-Onset): Symptoms appear between 6-18 months with moderate severity; individuals may sit unaided but struggle with standing or walking.
  - Type 3 (Juvenile-Onset): Milder form with onset after 18 months; affected individuals can often walk but may lose this ability over time.
  - Type 4 (Adult-Onset): Mildest form, typically with adult onset (usually after 30 years) and slower progression.
- Respiratory Issues: Due to weakened respiratory muscles, leading to increased infection risk and respiratory distress.
- Feeding and Swallowing Difficulties: Common in severe cases, especially in SMA Type 1.
- Joint Contractures and Scoliosis: Decreased mobility and muscle weakness contribute to skeletal complications.

- Intellectual Development: It is important to note that intellectual development is typically normal in SMA.

Genetic Diagnosis

- Genetic Testing for SMN1 Deletion or Mutation:
    - Quantitative PCR or MLPA to identify homozygous deletion of exon 7 of the SMN1 gene, which accounts for about 95% of SMA cases.
    - SMN1 gene sequencing to identify point mutations or deletions.
    - Copy number analysis to determine the number of SMN2 gene copies, which helps predict disease severity.
- Newborn Screening: Newborns are screened for changes in SMN genes to enable early intervention.

Genetic Counselling

- **Review of Medical and Family History**

  Obtain a detailed review of medical and developmental history, including hypotonia, delayed motor milestones, muscle weakness, and feeding or respiratory issues. A three-generation pedigree should be constructed to assess inheritance patterns and identify potential carriers. Document any history of unexplained infant deaths, neuromuscular conditions, or unexplained hypotonia in the family.

- **Discussion of Diagnosis**

  Explain that SMA results from a deficiency of the SMN protein due to homozygous loss of SMN1 function. The type of SMA correlates with the age of onset and, importantly, the number of SMN2 copies, which influences SMN protein production. A clear clinical explanation of motor neuron degeneration and its consequences and available treatments should be provided.

- **Inheritance Pattern and Recurrence Risk**

  SMA follows an autosomal recessive inheritance pattern. Parents of an affected child are typically asymptomatic carriers. When both parents are carriers, each pregnancy has a 25% risk of having an affected child, a 50% chance of being a carrier, and a 25% chance of being unaffected. Rare cases (2%) due to de novo mutations or parental germline mosaicism are possible and should be discussed as they impact recurrence risk.

- **Pre-test Counselling**

  Explain the purpose, benefits, and limitations of genetic testing for diagnosis, carrier status, or reproductive planning. Outline potential outcomes, including emotional implications and test limitations, such as undetected rare mutations. Discussion should facilitate informed decision-making for genetic testing based on the clinical context.

- **Post-test Counselling**

  Interpret the results and explain the findings. If a pathogenic mutation is identified in the SMN1 gene, the diagnosis of SMA is confirmed. The family should be informed of the specific SMN1 pathogenic variants, the SMN2 copy number (which has significant prognostic value and implications for therapy), and the available disease-modifying therapies. Cascade testing should be offered to extended family members to identify other carriers. If no mutation is detected despite strong clinical suspicion, additional testing (e.g., NGS) or muscle biopsy may be needed.

- **Medical Management and Surveillance**

  SMA requires multidisciplinary care involving neurology, pulmonology, orthopedics, and nutrition. Gene therapy (Onasemnogene abeparvovec) and SMN2 splicing modifiers (Nusinersen, Risdiplam) can modify disease progression. Supportive care includes respiratory support, physiotherapy, and nutritional and orthopedic management. Regular monitoring of scoliosis, contractures, respiratory function, and feeding issues is essential, with early intervention improving outcomes.

- **Reproductive and Family Planning**

  Discuss options like preimplantation genetic diagnosis (PGD) in conjunction with IVF to reduce transmission risk, or prenatal testing to identify SMA in utero. Explain alternatives such as gamete donation (sperm or egg) or adoption for families with a known risk, and provide information on their implications.

- **Psychosocial Support**

  Counselling should address the profound emotional toll of a chronic neurodegenerative condition, even with the advent of new therapies. Families may experience anticipatory grief, anxiety, guilt, and significant financial or caregiving strain. Referrals to support groups, psychologists, social workers, and palliative care specialists are recommended.

- **Follow-Up and Referrals**

  Schedule regular follow-up visits to monitor progression, support therapy adherence, and address emerging needs. Refer to specialists including neurologists, pulmonologists, gastroenterologists, physical therapists, occupational therapists, speech-language pathologists, orthopedists, and social workers, for comprehensive support.

- **Documentation**

  Thorough documentation should include pedigree, clinical findings, consent forms, genetic test reports, management plan, and family discussions. Records should be securely stored and updated periodically, especially as therapies and outcomes evolve.

References

1. Mercuri, E., et al. SMA Care Group (2018). Diagnosis and management of spinal muscular atrophy: Part 1: Recommendations for diagnosis, rehabilitation, orthopedic and nutritional care. Neuromuscular disorders : NMD, 28(2), 103–115.
2. Finkel, R. S., et al. SMA Care group (2018). Diagnosis and management of spinal muscular atrophy: Part 2: Pulmonary and acute care; medications, supplements and immunizations; other organ systems; and ethics. Neuromuscular disorders : NMD, 28(3), 197–207.
3. Nishio, H., Niba, E. T. E., Saito, T., Okamoto, K., Takeshima, Y., & Awano, H. (2023). Spinal Muscular Atrophy: The Past, Present, and Future of Diagnosis and Treatment. International journal of molecular sciences, 24(15), 11939.
4. Farrar, M. A., & Kiernan, M. C. (2015). The Genetics of Spinal Muscular Atrophy: Progress and Challenges. Neurotherapeutics : the journal of the American Society for Experimental NeuroTherapeutics, 12(2), 290–302.
5. Rouzier, C., Chaussenot, A., & Paquis-Flucklinger, V. (2020). Molecular diagnosis and genetic counseling for spinal muscular atrophy (SMA). Archives de Pédiatrie, 27(7), 7S9-7S14.

Congenital Adrenal Hyperplasia

Introduction

- Congenital Adrenal Hyperplasia (CAH) refers to a group of autosomal recessive disorders affecting adrenal steroid biosynthesis.
- The most common form is 21-hydroxylase deficiency, accounting for over 90% of cases.
- CAH affects both males and females and can present with salt-wasting crises, ambiguous genitalia, or later-onset symptoms.
- It is a potentially life-threatening but treatable condition with appropriate medical and genetic management.
- Newborn screening programs in many countries now routinely test for CAH.

Genetic Etiology

- 21-hydroxylase deficiency (21-OHD) accounts for more than 90% of CAH cases. This enzyme is crucial for the synthesis of cortisol and aldosterone from cholesterol.
- Mutations in the CYP21A2 gene, located in chromosome 6p21.3, leads to impaired 21-hydroxylase activity, resulting in deficient cortisol and aldosterone production, and consequently, a buildup of their precursors (e.g., 17-hydroxyprogesterone) that are shunted

towards the androgen synthesis pathway, leading to an excess of adrenal androgens.

- Reduced cortisol levels lead to a loss of negative feedback on the hypothalamic-pituitary-adrenal (HPA) axis. This results in the overstimulation of the adrenal gland by adrenocorticotropic hormone (ACTH) from the pituitary, causing adrenal hyperplasia (enlargement) and the overproduction of adrenal androgens.
- The severity of CAH depends on the specific mutation(s) in the CYP21A2 gene and the residual enzyme activity level, leading to a spectrum of clinical presentations, categorized into classic (severe) and non-classic (milder) forms.
- The CYP21A2 gene is located in a highly polymorphic region with a pseudogene (CYP21A1P), making molecular analysis complex due to the presence of common gene deletions, duplications, and conversions.

Clinical Manifestations

- Classic CAH (Severe):
  - Salt-wasting form: Presents in infancy with life-threatening adrenal crises, dehydration, hyponatremia, and hyperkalemia.
  - Simple virilizing form: Causes ambiguous genitalia in affected females at birth and progressive virilization (e.g., early pubic hair, accelerated growth) in both sexes.
- Non-classic CAH (Mild):
  - Later-onset symptoms include early puberty, acne, hirsutism, menstrual irregularities in females, and infertility.
  - Males may experience advanced growth but have normal genitalia at birth.

Genetic Diagnosis

- Hormonal Testing:
  - Newborn screening measures 17-hydroxyprogesterone (17-OHP) levels. Markedly elevated 17-OHP levels are indicative of 21-OHD CAH and require confirmatory testing.
- Molecular Testing of CYP21A2:
  - Genetic testing included DNA sequencing, deletion/duplication analysis to identify specific mutations or deletions in the CYP21A2 gene is the definitive method to confirm the diagnosis. It helps to categorize disease severity based on genotype-phenotype correlation, and aids in genetic counselling
  - Prenatal diagnosis for at-risk pregnancies can be performed via chorionic villus sampling (CVS) or amniocentesis to identify CYP21A2 mutations in the fetus.

Genetic Counselling

- **Review of Medical and Family History**

  Counselling begins with a thorough assessment of family history, focusing on unexplained neonatal deaths (especially males with normal genitalia), ambiguous genitalia, early virilization, infertility, or adrenal crises. A three-generation pedigree and consanguinity assessment should be documented. Details of sibling deaths or salt-wasting episodes are crucial in identifying autosomal recessive inheritance patterns and the severity of disease in the family.

- **Discussion of Diagnosis**

  The diagnosis of CAH should be explained in terms of defective steroid biosynthesis due to 21-hydroxylase deficiency. The counsellor should clarify the clinical spectrum from severe salt-wasting to non-classic forms and emphasize the impact on adrenal function and sexual development. The link between genotype and phenotype variability should also be addressed during discussion.

- **Inheritance Pattern and Recurrence Risk**

  CAH is inherited in an autosomal recessive manner. When both parents are carriers, each child has a 25% chance of being affected, 50% chance of being a carrier, and 25% chance of being unaffected. Counsellors should explain the significance of compound heterozygous mutations and outline recurrence risks for future pregnancies.

- **Pre-test Counselling**

  Before testing, informed consent should be obtained with a clear explanation of the test purpose, methodology, limitations, and implications. For carrier testing and prenatal diagnosis, the emotional, ethical, and reproductive implications should be discussed. The couple should be aware of the possibility of incidental findings and the need for genetic confirmation in asymptomatic siblings.

- **Post-test Counselling**

  Communicate genetic test results, explaining positive, negative, or carrier status for individuals and their family members. Discuss the clinical implications of the specific CYP21A2 mutations identified, the expected disease severity, and management strategies. Provide family screening recommendations and cascade testing as appropriate for at-risk relatives.

- **Medical Management and Surveillance**

  Review lifelong management strategies, including chronic glucocorticoid replacement therapy to normalize ACTH and suppress androgen excess, and mineralocorticoid replacement therapy for salt-wasting forms. Regular monitoring for growth, bone age, electrolyte levels, blood pressure, and androgen levels is crucial to optimize treatment, prevent complications (e.g., adrenal crisis, virilization, short stature, obesity), and improve long-term outcomes.

- **Reproductive and Family Planning**

  Discuss reproductive options for at-risk couples such as preimplantation genetic diagnosis (PGD) in conjunction with in vitro fertilization (IVF) to prevent CAH in offspring. Prenatal diagnosis via CVS or amniocentesis can also be performed if parents are known carriers. For affected individuals, discuss the impact of CAH on fertility and the need for ongoing management. Outline alternatives such as gamete donation (sperm or egg) or adoption for couples who wish to avoid transmitting the genetic condition.

- **Psychosocial Support**

  Provide resources for coping with a chronic illness, including support groups, and mental health resources. Offer information on managing challenges related to gender identity (especially in individuals born with ambiguous genitalia), body image, sexual health, and long-term adherence to medication and monitoring.

- **Follow-Up and Referrals**

  Schedule regular follow-up visits to assess treatment efficacy, monitor health, and address emerging needs. Refer to a multidisciplinary team of specialists, including endocrinologists, geneticists, mental health professionals, and social workers for comprehensive and coordinated care.

- **Documentation**

  Comprehensive documentation should include the family history, counselling notes, informed consent for testing, genetic test results, and management plans. Counselling summaries should record the diagnosis, risks, options discussed, referrals made, and follow-up recommendations. Records should be stored securely with provisions for confidentiality.

References

1. Merke, D. P., & Auchus, R. J. (2020). Congenital Adrenal Hyperplasia Due to 21-Hydroxylase Deficiency. The New England journal of medicine, 383(13), 1248–1261.
2. Speiser, P. W., et al (2018). Congenital Adrenal Hyperplasia Due to Steroid 21-Hydroxylase Deficiency: An Endocrine Society Clinical Practice Guideline. The Journal of clinical endocrinology and metabolism, 103(11), 4043–4088.
3. Krone, N., & Arlt, W. (2009). Genetics of congenital adrenal hyperplasia. Best practice & research. Clinical endocrinology & metabolism, 23(2), 181–192.
4. Finkielstain, G. P., Vieites, A., Bergadá, I., & Rey, R. A. (2021). Disorders of Sex Development of Adrenal Origin. Frontiers in endocrinology, 12, 770782.

X-LINKED RECESSIVE DISORDERS

List of X-Linked recessive disorders

Hemophilia A and B	G6PD Deficiency
Duchenne Muscular Dystrophy (DMD)	Lesch-Nyhan Syndrome
Becker Muscular Dystrophy (BMD)	Fabry's disease
Color Blindness (Red/Green)	Hunter Syndrome
Adrenoleukodystrophy (ALD)	X-Linked Agammaglobulinemia (XLA)
OTC Deficiency	Diabetes insipidus (nephrogenic type)

General characteristics of X-Linked recessive inheritance pattern

- In X-linked recessive disorders, females must inherit two copies of the mutated gene (one from each parent) to be affected, whereas males only need one mutated gene on their single X chromosome to express the condition.
- Hence, males are predominantly affected, and females are typically carriers.

- When the mother is a carrier and the father is unaffected, each male child has a 50% chance of being affected, while each female child has a 50% chance of being a carrier.
- Carrier females typically do not exhibit symptoms (are asymptomatic) due to the presence of a second, normal X chromosome, although mild symptoms can occasionally occur due to skewed X-inactivation.
- If the father is affected, all daughters will be carriers (obligate carriers), but none of the sons will inherit the disorder (i.e., no male-to-male transmission).
- Consanguinity is not typically a significant factor in X-linked recessive inheritance, but can increase the frequency of carriers in the population.
- Males are predominantly affected since they have only one X chromosome. Females are less frequently affected only if both parents contribute a mutated gene or if X-inactivation skews expression.
- Variable expressivity in carriers: Carrier females may exhibit mild symptoms due to random nature of X-inactivation, which can lead to variable expressivity of phenotype.

Hemophilia

Introduction

- Hemophilia is a group of X-linked recessive bleeding disorders characterized by a deficiency or dysfunction of clotting factors.
- The two main types are Hemophilia A (factor VIII deficiency) and Hemophilia B (factor IX deficiency).
- Hemophilia primarily affects males, while females are typically carriers.
- It leads to prolonged bleeding, spontaneous hemorrhages, and joint damage if not adequately managed.

Genetic Etiology

- Hemophilia is caused by mutations in genes responsible for producing clotting factors, which are critical for blood clot formation.
- Hemophilia A (Factor VIII deficiency, more common, accounting for approximately 80-85% of cases) is caused by mutations in the F8 gene on the Xq28 chromosome, which encodes factor VIII.
- Hemophilia B (Factor IX deficiency, less common, accounting for approximately 15-20% of cases) is caused by mutations in the F9 gene on Xq27.1, which encodes factor IX.
- A deficiency or dysfunction in either factor VIII or IX disrupts the intrinsic pathway of the coagulation cascade, leading to impaired

fibrin clot formation, prolonged bleeding, and increased risk of spontaneous bleeding episodes.

Clinical Manifestations

- Frequent and Prolonged Bleeding: Bleeding episodes may occur after injury or surgery, and in severe cases, spontaneously without apparent cause.
- Joint and Muscle Bleeding (Hemarthrosis): Common in severe hemophilia, leading to joint pain, swelling, and potential long-term joint damage if untreated.
- Easy Bruising and Hematomas: Minor traumas can lead to significant bruising or deep tissue bleeding.
- Bleeding after Dental Work or Surgery: Bleeding may be difficult to control and can pose significant health risks.
- Intracranial Hemorrhage: A serious and potentially life-threatening complication, especially in severe hemophilia, that can lead to neurological damage or death.
- Gastrointestinal and Urogenital Bleeding: Can occur spontaneously or after minor trauma, leading to significant blood loss.
- Severity Variability: Severity is classified as mild, moderate, or severe, based on basal clotting factor activity levels.

  Severe hemophilia: Factor activity <1% of normal. Often presents in infancy with spontaneous bleeding (joints, muscles, intracranial).

  Moderate hemophilia: Factor activity 1-5% of normal. Bleeding typically occurs after mild trauma or surgery, with occasional spontaneous bleeds.

  Mild hemophilia: Factor activity 5-40% of normal. Bleeding usually occurs only after significant trauma, surgery, or dental procedures. May only be identified in adolescence or adulthood.

Genetic Diagnosis

- Clotting Factor Assays: Measure factor VIII or IX activity in blood to determine hemophilia type and severity.
- Genetic Testing for F8 or F9 Mutations: This is the definitive diagnostic method. It confirms diagnosis, identifies specific pathogenic mutations (e.g., intron 22 inversion, intron 1 inversion in F8 which are common; point mutations, deletions, insertions in both genes), and is crucial for accurate carrier testing, prenatal diagnosis, and genetic counselling.
- Carrier Testing: Females in families with a history of hemophilia can be tested to determine carrier status, especially for family planning purposes. This is ideally done by identifying the specific familial mutation.
- Activated Partial Thromboplastin Time (aPTT): This coagulation screening test is typically prolonged in hemophilia A and B, serving as an initial indicator, though it does not specify the deficient factor or severity.

Genetic Counselling

- **Review of Medical and Family History**

  A detailed personal and family history should be obtained, focusing on bleeding episodes, history of excessive bruising, hemarthrosis, or surgical complications. A three-generation pedigree should be drawn, noting affected males, carrier females, consanguinity, and history of spontaneous miscarriages or neonatal deaths. Inquire about specific bleeding challenges for females in the family, such as heavy periods or postpartum hemorrhage.
- **Discussion of Diagnosis**

  Explain the genetic basis and X-linked inheritance pattern of hemophilia. Inform patients that male offspring of carrier mothers are at risk, while female offspring may be carriers. Provide an overview of clinical manifestations based on factor deficiency type (VIII or IX) and severity, including the potential for spontaneous and severe bleeding episodes.

- **Inheritance Pattern and Recurrence Risk**

  Hemophilia is X-linked recessive, so male children of carrier mothers have a 50% chance of being affected, while female children have a 50% chance of being carriers. Emphasize that affected fathers cannot pass the condition to sons but will pass the gene to all daughters, making them obligate carriers. Explain the phenomenon of X-inactivation and how skewed X-inactivation can rarely lead to mild symptoms in carrier females.

- **Pre-test Counselling**

  Explain the purpose, benefits, and implications of genetic testing for confirming hemophilia type, identifying carriers, and guiding future pregnancies. Discuss the emotional, social, and reproductive considerations related to knowing one's carrier or affected status. Emphasize the importance of early diagnosis for prompt management. Obtain informed consent prior to genetic testing.

- **Post-test Counselling**

  Provide a clear interpretation of genetic test results, explaining positive, negative, and carrier statuses for family members. If positive, discuss the risk of hemophilia for future generations. Offer family screening for siblings and other relatives who may be at risk of being carriers or affected. Carrier females with low factor levels should be informed of their personal bleeding risks and the need for appropriate management.

- **Medical Management and Surveillance**

  Review treatment options, such as factor replacement therapy (either factor VIII or IX) for bleeding prevention and management. Emphasize the importance of regular follow-up with a hematologist and prophylactic care to prevent joint damage, especially in severe cases. Advise on safe lifestyle modifications, including avoiding high-impact activities to reduce injury risk, and recommend prompt treatment for any signs of bleeding.

- **Reproductive and Family Planning**

  Discuss family planning options, including preimplantation genetic diagnosis (PGD) in conjunction with in vitro fertilization (IVF) to avoid passing on hemophilia to offspring. Explain prenatal testing options like chorionic villus sampling (CVS) and amniocentesis for at-risk pregnancies if parents are known carriers. Discuss reproductive alternatives such as gamete donation or adoption.

- **Psychosocial Support**

  Offer support for coping with the physical, emotional, and psychological impacts of managing a lifelong bleeding disorder. Provide resources for accessing support groups and connecting with other families affected by hemophilia. Address any fears or concerns about passing the disorder to future generations and provide emotional support for dealing with social implications, including school/work accommodations.

- **Follow-Up and Referrals**

  Schedule regular follow-up visits for monitoring and managing hemophilia. Refer to specialists as needed, including hematologists, orthopedic surgeons, physical therapists, pain management specialists, and geneticists, for comprehensive and coordinated care. Female carriers may need gynecological referrals for heavy menstruation management.

- **Documentation**

  Comprehensive documentation should include the family pedigree, clinical findings, informed consent for testing, genetic test results with interpretations, and a summary of counselling discussions and the proposed management plan. Details of specialist referrals and follow-up schedules should also be recorded. All records must be securely stored, ensuring confidentiality and access only by authorized personnel.

References

1. Srivastava A, Santagostino E, Dougall A, et al. WFH Guidelines for the Management of Hemophilia, 3rd edition. Haemophilia : the official journal of the World Federation of Hemophilia, 26 Suppl 6, 1–158.
2. Peyvandi, F., Garagiola, I., & Young, G. (2016). The past and future of haemophilia: diagnosis, treatments, and its complications. Lancet (London, England), 388(10040), 187–197.
3. Bolton-Maggs PHB, Pasi KJ. Haemophilias A and B. Lancet. 2003;361(9371):1801-1809.
4. De Wolf, D., Singh, K., Chuah, M. K., & VandenDriessche, T. (2023). Hemophilia Gene Therapy: The End of the Beginning?. Human gene therapy, 34(17-18), 782–792.

Duchenne Muscular Dystrophy

Introduction

- Duchenne Muscular Dystrophy (DMD) is a severe X-linked recessive neuromuscular disorder.
- It primarily affects boys, with onset in early childhood.
- Characterized by progressive muscle weakness, loss of ambulation, and premature death due to respiratory or cardiac failure.
- DMD has a significant psychosocial and reproductive impact on families, necessitating genetic counselling.

Genetic Etiology

- DMD is caused by pathogenic mutations in the DMD gene located on the Xp21.2 chromosome, which encodes dystrophin, a protein essential for muscle cell stability and function. These mutations result in a frameshift or nonsense mutation, leading to the absence or severe truncation of functional dystrophin protein.
- Becker Muscular Dystrophy (BMD) is a milder form of DMD with later onset. It is also caused by mutations in the DMD gene, but these mutations result in an in-frame deletion or duplication, allowing for the production of a partially functional dystrophin protein.

- The absence or severe deficiency of functional dystrophin compromises the integrity of the sarcolemma, making muscle fibers highly susceptible to damage during contraction.
- This leads to progressive muscle fiber necrosis, inflammation, and replacement of muscle tissue by fibrous and adipose tissue, resulting in muscle weakness, loss of motor abilities, and ultimately, severe cardiopulmonary complications.
- Due to the X-linked recessive inheritance, males with a DMD gene mutation are affected, while females are usually asymptomatic carriers, though they may have some clinical manifestations (mild muscle weakness or cardiomyopathy)

Clinical Manifestations

- Early Muscle Weakness: Symptoms often appear between ages 2-5, starting in the proximal muscles (hips and shoulders), causing difficulty in activities like walking, running, or climbing stairs. Initial signs may include a waddling gait and frequent falls.
- Gower's Sign: A classic feature where children use their hands to push off from their knees to stand due to weak hip and thigh muscles.
- Pseudohypertrophy of Calves: Enlargement of calf muscles due to replacement of muscle tissue with fat and connective tissue, despite muscle weakness.
- Progressive Weakness and Loss of Ambulation: As the disease progresses, affected individuals lose the ability to walk, typically requiring a wheelchair by ages 10-14.
- Cardiomyopathy and Respiratory Complications: Progressive involvement of heart and respiratory muscles leads to complications, often becoming life-threatening by late teens or early adulthood.
- Cognitive Impairment: Some children may experience mild intellectual disability due to dystrophin's role in brain function.

Genetic Diagnosis

- CK (Creatine Kinase) Test: Elevated CK levels in blood indicate muscle damage, commonly seen in DMD.
- Serum creatine kinase levels show "100 fold" increase in DMD and "50 fold" increase in BMD. Normal CK levels are generally below 200 IU/L.
- Genetic Testing for DMD Mutations: Confirms diagnosis by detecting mutations in the DMD gene, aiding in family planning and risk assessment for relatives.
- Deletion/duplication events which accounts for 60-70% of DMD is identified by MLPA or chromosomal microarray. DNA sequencing is used for detection of point mutations, small insertions/deletions, and splice site variants.
- Carrier Testing and Prenatal Diagnosis: Female relatives can undergo genetic testing to determine carrier status. Prenatal testing (chorionic villus sampling or amniocentesis) can be done for pregnancies at risk if a familial DMD mutation is known.

Genetic Counselling

- **Review of Medical and Family History**

  A three-generation pedigree should be meticulously collected to identify other affected males and potential female carriers. Document history of muscle weakness, developmental motor delays, early loss of ambulation, cardiomyopathy, respiratory issues, or unexplained elevated CK levels in family members. Consanguinity and previous pregnancy losses should also be assessed. It's important to ask about female relatives with muscle weakness, cardiomyopathy, or elevated CK levels, as they may be symptomatic carriers.

- **Discussion of Diagnosis**

  Explain the genetic cause, X-linked recessive inheritance pattern, and the progressive nature of DMD. Emphasize that males with the mutation will develop the disease, while female carriers generally show no or very mild symptoms, although they are at a lifelong risk for dilated cardiomyopathy (DCM) and may have muscle cramps or fatigue.

- **Inheritance Pattern**

  DMD follows an X-linked recessive inheritance pattern. A carrier mother has a 50% chance of passing the mutated gene to each child. Sons who inherit the mutation will be affected, while daughters who inherit it will be carriers. Affected fathers cannot pass the condition to their sons but will pass the gene to all their daughters, making them obligate carriers. Discuss the possibility of germline mosaicism in the mother, where the mutation is present only in her germ cells, leading to an affected child despite the mother testing negative in somatic cells. Discuss the possibility of de novo mutations occurring in the affected male (accounting for 30% of cases), where neither parent is a carrier.

- **Pre-test Counselling**

  Discuss the purpose and implications of genetic testing, including diagnosis, carrier detection, and reproductive planning. Address potential emotional and psychological concerns related to a diagnosis, carrier status, and the progressive nature of the disease. Informed consent must be obtained before genetic testing.

- **Post-test Counselling**

  Explain test results clearly, addressing positive, negative, or carrier statuses and their implications for family members. For affected individuals, discuss the specific mutation type and its relevance for potential gene-specific therapies. Recommend carrier testing for at-risk female relatives and facilitate appropriate cardiac surveillance. Negative or inconclusive results should be explained carefully, considering technical limitations and the possibility of germline mosaicism.

- **Medical Management and Surveillance**

  Review multidisciplinary management involving regular follow-ups with neurology, cardiology, pulmonology, physical therapy, occupational therapy, and nutrition specialists. Treatment options include corticosteroids to slow disease progression, physical therapy and orthopedic support for managing contractures and scoliosis, and management of respiratory and cardiac complications. Highlight availability of exon skipping drugs and gene therapy. Emphasize the importance of monitoring respiratory function and heart health, as these are often affected and crucial for survival.

- **Reproductive and Family Planning**

  Discuss reproductive options for at-risk couples. These include preimplantation genetic diagnosis (PGD) in conjunction with in vitro fertilization (IVF) to avoid passing DMD to offspring. Offer information on prenatal diagnosis (CVS or amniocentesis) for carriers considering pregnancy. Outline alternatives such as gamete donation or adoption for families who wish to avoid transmitting the genetic condition.

- **Psychosocial Support**

  Offer counselling to address the profound emotional impact of a DMD diagnosis, including coping with progressive disability, loss of function, chronic pain, and planning for future care. Provide resources to connect with support groups and other families affected by DMD. Address grief, anxiety, and depression that may arise in affected individuals and their families.

- **Follow-Up and Referrals**

  Schedule regular follow-up visits for ongoing support, surveillance, and management. Refer to a specialized multidisciplinary team, including neurologists, cardiologists, pulmonologists, physical therapists, occupational therapists, speech-language pathologists, orthopedists, nutritionists, and mental health professionals to ensure comprehensive care.

- **Documentation**

  Detailed documentation should include the pedigree, clinical summary, informed consent for testing, genetic test reports, and a summary of counselling discussions. Records must be stored securely, ensuring patient confidentiality and access by authorized personnel only.

References

1. Birnkrant, D. J., et al & DMD Care Considerations Working Group (2018). Diagnosis and management of Duchenne muscular dystrophy, part 1: diagnosis, and neuromuscular, rehabilitation, endocrine, and gastrointestinal and nutritional management. The Lancet. Neurology, 17(3), 251–267.
2. Birnkrant, D. J., et al & DMD Care Considerations Working Group (2018). Diagnosis and management of Duchenne muscular dystrophy, part 2: respiratory, cardiac, bone health, and orthopaedic management. The Lancet. Neurology, 17(4), 347–361.
3. Mah J. K. (2016). Current and emerging treatment strategies for Duchenne muscular dystrophy. Neuropsychiatric disease and treatment, 12, 1795–1807.
4. Grimm, T., Kress, W., Meng, G., & Müller, C. R. (2012). Risk assessment and genetic counseling in families with Duchenne muscular dystrophy. Acta myologica : myopathies and cardiomyopathies : official journal of the Mediterranean Society of Myology, 31(3), 179–183.
5. Pickart, A. M., et al. (2025). Genetic counseling for the dystrophinopathies-Practice resource of the National Society of Genetic Counselors. Journal of genetic counseling, 34(1), e1892.

G6PD Deficiency

Introduction

- G6PD deficiency is one of the most common enzymopathies worldwide, affecting over 400 million people.
- It is a hereditary red blood cell disorder that that affects red blood cell stability, leading to their premature destruction (hemolysis) under oxidative stress.
- Most individuals are asymptomatic until exposed to triggers such as certain drugs, infections, or foods.
- Genetic counselling is essential for early identification, risk communication, and preventive education in families.

Genetic Etiology

- Glucose-6-Phosphate Dehydrogenase (G6PD) Deficiency is an X-linked recessive metabolic disorder
- G6PD deficiency is caused by mutations in the G6PD gene, located on the Xq28 chromosome, which encodes the enzyme glucose-6-phosphate dehydrogenase.
- This enzyme is crucial for the pentose phosphate pathway (PPP), specifically for generating NADPH (Nicotinamide Adenine Dinucleotide Phosphate, reduced form). NADPH is vital for protecting

red blood cells from oxidative damage by reducing glutathione, a key antioxidant.

- The deficiency of G6PD enzyme impairs the RBC's ability to produce sufficient NADPH. Without adequate NADPH, the RBCs cannot effectively reduce harmful reactive oxygen species (ROS) and repair oxidative damage.
- This leads to the accumulation of oxidized hemoglobin and increased oxidative stress, which causes the red blood cell membrane to become rigid and fragile, leading to premature destruction in response to certain triggers like infections, medications, and specific foods.

Clinical Manifestations

- Hemolytic Anemia: Patients with G6PD deficiency may experience episodes of hemolytic anemia, characterized by symptoms such as fatigue, pallor, jaundice, dark urine, and back pain.
- Neonatal Jaundice: G6PD-deficient newborns have an increased risk of jaundice in the first few days after birth, which may require treatment to prevent complications.
- Favism: Acute hemolysis may occur after the ingestion of fava beans or exposure to certain drugs, resulting in rapid anemia.
- Chronic Hemolysis: Some individuals may experience chronic low-level hemolysis without overt symptoms, though this is less common.

Genetic Diagnosis

- G6PD Enzyme Assay: This test measures G6PD enzyme activity in red blood cells and is the primary test to confirm the diagnosis of G6PD deficiency.
- Genetic Testing: DNA-based testing to identify mutations in G6PD gene can confirm the specific mutation, which may be helpful in populations with known G6PD variants and to assess carrier status in females, as enzyme assays may be less sensitive in carriers.

Genetic Counselling

- **Review of Medical and Family History**

  Collect a detailed three-generation family history along with consanguinity information, focusing on episodes of anemia, unexplained neonatal jaundice, or hemolytic episodes after exposure to certain drugs, foods, or infections. Ascertain geographical ancestry, as G6PD deficiency is highly prevalent in certain populations from malarial regions

- **Discussion of Diagnosis**

  Explain G6PD deficiency, its X-linked recessive inheritance pattern, and the biochemical basis of hemolytic episodes. Symptoms typically occur after exposure to specific triggers. Emphasize that many individuals remain asymptomatic until exposed to such triggers. Describe how the condition predominantly affects males, while females may be carriers with typically milder or no symptoms, but some carriers can experience symptomatic hemolysis due to skewed X-inactivation.

- **Inheritance Pattern**

  As an X-linked recessive disorder, male children of carrier mothers have a 50% chance of being affected, while female children have a 50% chance of being carriers. Affected fathers will pass the gene to all daughters (who will be carriers) but not to sons. Discuss the possibility of de novo mutations and germline mosaicism.

- **Pre-test Counselling**

  Discuss the importance and limitations of genetic testing for carrier detection, particularly in females, and the value of enzyme assays in determining deficiency. Informed consent should be obtained prior to genetic testing. Address any emotional concerns about carrier status and its impact on personal health and family planning.

- **Post-test Counselling**

  Communicate test results clearly and explain the implications of positive, negative, or carrier statuses. For affected individuals or carriers, discuss personalized risk management strategies, including a comprehensive list of substances to avoid. Recommend cascade testing for at-risk family members, especially females who may be carriers.

- **Medical Management and Surveillance**

  Emphasize avoiding known triggers of hemolysis, such as fava beans, certain medications (e.g., sulfonamides, antimalarials), and infections. Educate patients and caregivers about early signs of hemolysis (dark urine, jaundice, fatigue) and advise immediate medical attention if symptoms occur. In cases of acute hemolysis, management may involve supportive care, including hydration, oxygen therapy, monitoring of hemoglobin levels, and potentially blood transfusions in severe cases.

- **Reproductive and Family Planning**

  Discuss reproductive options for carriers or affected individuals, including preimplantation genetic diagnosis (PGD) in conjunction with in vitro fertilization (IVF), and prenatal testing (chorionic villus sampling or amniocentesis) if parents are known carriers and decide to pursue it. Discuss the specific risks and considerations for male and female offspring. Outline alternatives such as gamete donation or adoption for families who wish to avoid transmitting the genetic condition.

- **Psychosocial Support**

  Provide resources for educational and support groups focused on G6PD deficiency. Offer counselling to address concerns about managing the condition, especially when faced with dietary and lifestyle restrictions, and the anxiety associated with avoiding triggers. Emphasize that most individuals with G6PD deficiency can lead normal lives with proper management.

- **Follow-Up and Referrals**

  Schedule follow-up appointments as needed, particularly after a hemolytic episode, to monitor for recovery and ensure compliance with lifestyle recommendations. Provide referrals to hematologists for definitive diagnosis and management, and to dietitians and physicians for detailed guidance on dietary and medication avoidance.

- **Documentation**

  All counselling sessions should be documented, including family history, informed consent, test results, discussion points, and follow-up plans. Pedigree charts and laboratory reports must be securely stored with appropriate confidentiality measures.

References

1. Cappellini MD, Fiorelli G. Glucose-6-phosphate dehydrogenase deficiency. *Lancet*. 2008;371(9606):64-74.
2. Luzzatto, L., Ally, M., & Notaro, R. (2020). Glucose-6-phosphate dehydrogenase deficiency. Blood, 136(11), 1225–1240.
3. Minucci, A., Moradkhani, K., Hwang, M. J., Zuppi, C., Giardina, B., & Capoluongo, E. (2012). Glucose-6-phosphate dehydrogenase (G6PD) mutations database: review of the "old" and update of the new mutations. Blood cells, molecules & diseases, 48(3), 154–165.
4. Frank J. E. (2005). Diagnosis and management of G6PD deficiency. American family physician, 72(7), 1277–1282.

X-LINKED DOMINANT DISORDERS

List of X-Linked dominant disorders

Vitamin D Resistant Rickets	Alport syndrome
Rett Syndrome	Incontinentia Pigmenti
Fragile X syndrome	Goltz Syndrome
CHILD Syndrome	X-Linked Dominant Charcot-Marie-Tooth

General characteristics of X-Linked dominant inheritance pattern

- In X-linked dominant disorders, a single copy of the mutated gene on the X chromosome can cause the disorder in both males and females. However, males often present with more severe symptoms due to having only one X chromosome (hemizygous).
- An affected father will pass the mutated gene to all daughters, who will be affected, but none of his sons will inherit the disorder. No male-to-male transmission.
- When the mother is affected, each child has a 50% chance of inheriting the mutation, regardless of sex. Thus, both male and female children have an equal probability of being affected.

- X-linked dominant disorders often show more severe symptoms in males than in females.
- Males can experience severe forms of the disorder, sometimes resulting in prenatal or early lethality, as seen in some X-linked dominant disorders.
- Females may exhibit variable expressivity due to random X-inactivation, where the mutated gene may not be expressed in all cells.
- The disorder is vertically transmitted and can appear in every generation, affecting both genders. However, daughters of affected fathers will always be affected.
- No skipping of generations is observed (unless there is reduced penetrance, which is less common for "dominant" patterns).
- Consanguinity is not a significant factor in the inheritance pattern, as a single dominant allele is sufficient to cause the disorder.

Fragile X Syndrome

Introduction

- Fragile X Syndrome (FXS) is the most common inherited cause of intellectual disability and a known monogenic cause of autism spectrum disorder.
- It primarily affects males but can also present with variable symptoms in females.
- Early diagnosis is crucial for timely interventions, education planning, and family support.
- Genetic counselling plays a key role in guiding families through diagnosis, inheritance patterns, and reproductive risk management.

Genetic Etiology

- Fragile X Syndrome (FXS) is an X-linked disorder
- FXS is caused by an unstable expansion of the CGG trinucleotide repeat in the 5' untranslated region of the FMR1 gene, located on the Xq27.3 chromosome.
- When the CGG repeats exceed 200 (full mutation), the region becomes hypermethylated, leading to transcriptional silencing of the gene. This results in a lack or severe deficiency of fragile X mental retardation protein (FMRP), which is critical for normal synaptic function, plasticity, and brain development.

- Individuals with an intermediate number of CGG repeats (55–200) are considered premutation carriers. These individuals may not show symptoms of full FXS but are at increased risk for Fragile X-associated Tremor/Ataxia Syndrome (FXTAS) in older men and, less commonly, in older women, and Fragile X-associated Primary Ovarian Insufficiency (FXPOI) in women. They may also experience other FMR1-associated conditions like anxiety or depression.
- The term "X-linked dominant" can be misleading because carrier females are often less severely affected than males, and some may be asymptomatic. Hence, it is an X-linked disorder with incomplete penetrance and variable expressivity, particularly in females

Clinical Manifestations

- Intellectual Disability: Ranges from mild to severe, more commonly affecting males. Many individuals with FXS have delays in speech and motor skills.
- Behavioural and Emotional Issues: Symptoms include hyperactivity, social anxiety, sensitivity to sensory stimuli, repetitive speech, poor eye contact, and hand flapping.
- Physical Features: Males with FXS may exhibit a long face, large ears, hyperextensible joints, flat feet, mitral valve prolapse, and macroorchidism (enlarged testes) post-puberty.
- Females with FXS: Often show milder symptoms due to the presence of a second, unaffected X chromosome. Symptoms in females may include learning disabilities, social anxiety, and mood disorders.

Genetic Diagnosis

- Molecular Testing for CGG Repeat Expansion: DNA testing and methylation analysis of the FMR1 gene identifies the CGG repeat number, confirming the diagnosis and differentiating between full mutation (>200 CGG repeats), premutation (55-200 CGG repeats), grey zone (45-54 CGG repeats) and normal alleles (< 45 CGG repeats).

- Carrier Testing: Female relatives can be tested to determine their carrier status, which is essential for family planning and understanding the risk of transmission to future generations.

Genetic Counselling

- **Review of Medical and Family History**

  Gather a detailed three-generation family history along with consanguinity information focusing on signs of intellectual disability, delayed speech, learning difficulties, autism spectrum behaviours, seizures, or related FMR1-associated syndromes like FXTAS and FXPOI. This is crucial as FXS often has a complex family history.

- **Discussion of Diagnosis**

  Explain the genetic cause of FXS, its X-linked inheritance pattern with incomplete penetrance and variable expressivity. Describe how the CGG expansion impacts FMR1 gene expression and FMRP production, leading to the range of cognitive, behavioural, and physical symptoms seen in FXS. Emphasize the implications for both males and females with the full mutation or premutation.

- **Inheritance Pattern and Recurrence Risk**

  Affected females with full mutation can be carriers and typically have milder symptoms, while affected males with full mutation often show more severe manifestations. Female carriers have a 50% chance of passing the mutation to each child regardless of sex, with sons often showing more severe symptoms. Affected males have intellectual disability and generally do not reproduce.

  From a female premutation carrier, the CGG repeat can expand to a full mutation when passed from a mother to her child, especially if the mother has a larger premutation allele. From a male premutation carrier, the CGG repeat in does not expand when passed to their daughters (expansion only occurs through female gametogenesis). They will only pass on their premutation allele. Therefore, all daughters of a male premutation carrier will inherit the premutation and be carriers.

Anticipation: Explain that the severity of the disorder and the age of onset may appear earlier in subsequent generations, due to the expansion of the CGG repeat size when transmitted through a female.

- **Pre-test Counselling**

  Discuss the purpose, benefits, and limitations of genetic testing, including its ability to confirm diagnosis, identify premutation carriers, and its implications for reproductive planning. Address potential emotional and psychological concerns related to learning about one's own or a family member's mutation/carrier status, and the implications for siblings and extended family. Obtain informed consent prior to genetic testing.

- **Post-test Counselling**

  Communicate test results and explain the implications of normal, intermediate, premutation, or full mutation status, including potential health implications (e.g., FXTAS, FXPOI) for family members. Offer recommendations for cascade testing for at-risk family members, especially females in the maternal lineage, to inform family planning and ongoing health surveillance.

- **Medical Management and Surveillance**

  Emphasize early intervention therapies, such as speech-language therapy, occupational therapy, physical therapy, and behavioural therapy, to optimize outcomes in individuals with FXS. Behavioural therapies and medications can help manage symptoms like anxiety, hyperactivity, attention deficits, and aggression. Monitor for any related health conditions, such as seizures, sleep disorders, gastrointestinal issues, FXTAS in older male carriers, and FXPOI in female carriers. Refer to specialists including, neurologists, mental health professionals, endocrinologists, cardiologists for multidisciplinary care.

- **Reproductive and Family Planning**

  Discuss reproductive options for premutation carriers or families with a known history of FXS, including preimplantation genetic diagnosis (PGD) in conjunction with in vitro fertilization (IVF) to select embryos without the full mutation. Offer information on prenatal diagnosis by chorionic villus sampling (CVS) or amniocentesis for pregnancies at risk. Discuss the possibility of adopting or using donor gametes.

- **Psychosocial Support**

  Offer resources for support groups, advocacy organizations, and educational materials to help families connect with others affected by FXS and access relevant resources. Address any concerns regarding coping with the emotional and social aspects of the condition, including challenges with daily living, educational planning, and long-term care.

- **Follow-Up and Referrals**

  Schedule follow-up visits to monitor the individual's progress, adjust therapies, and address new questions or needs. Provide referrals to pediatricians, neurologists, geneticists, psychologists/psychiatrists, speech/occupational/physical therapists, and other support services to ensure multidisciplinary care.

- **Documentation**

  Documentation must include a complete family history, informed consent, genetic test results, discussion summaries, and follow-up recommendations. All records should be maintained securely, and cascade testing efforts must be recorded for future reference.

References

1. Hagerman RJ, Hagerman PJ. *Fragile X Syndrome: Diagnosis, Treatment, and Research.* 4th ed. The Johns Hopkins University Press; 2015.
2. Sherman, S., Pletcher, B. A., & Driscoll, D. A. (2005). Fragile X syndrome: diagnostic and carrier testing. Genetics in medicine : official journal of the American College of Medical Genetics, 7(8), 584–587.
3. Monaghan, K. G., et al. (2013). ACMG Standards and Guidelines for fragile X testing: a revision to the disease-specific supplements to the Standards and Guidelines for Clinical Genetics Laboratories of the American College of Medical Genetics and Genomics. Genetics in medicine : official journal of the American College of Medical Genetics, 15(7), 575–586.
4. McConkie-Rosell, A., Finucane, B., Cronister, A., Abrams, L., Bennett, R. L., & Pettersen, B. J. (2005). Genetic counseling for fragile x syndrome: updated recommendations of the national society of genetic counselors. Journal of genetic counseling, 14(4), 249–270.
5. Finucane, B., Abrams, L., Cronister, A., Archibald, A. D., Bennett, R. L., & McConkie-Rosell, A. (2012). Genetic counseling and testing for FMR1 gene mutations: practice guidelines of the national society of genetic counselors. Journal of genetic counseling, 21(6), 752–760.

X-linked hypophosphatemia

Introduction

- Vitamin D-Resistant Rickets (VDRR) is a group of hereditary disorders characterized by impaired phosphate metabolism and defective bone mineralization.
- The most common form is X-linked hypophosphatemic rickets (XLH).
- Affected individuals present with rickets-like symptoms despite adequate vitamin D levels.
- Genetic counselling plays a critical role in diagnosis, inheritance assessment, and reproductive planning.

Genetic Etiology

- X-linked hypophosphatemic rickets (XLH), is an X-linked dominant disorder characterized by impaired renal phosphate reabsorption, leading to chronic hypophosphatemia and defective bone mineralization
- XLH is primarily caused by mutations in the PHEX gene (Phosphate-regulating gene with homologies to Endopeptidases on the X chromosome) located on the Xp22.1 chromosome. This gene mutation disrupts phosphate regulation in the kidneys, leading to excessive phosphate loss, which is crucial for bone and dental health.

- The PHEX gene mutation leads to an excess production and/or reduced degradation of Fibroblast Growth Factor 23 (FGF23). Elevated FGF23 reduces renal phosphate reabsorption and inhibits 1α-hydroxylase, thereby reducing calcitriol production. This leads to hypophosphatemia, impaired intestinal calcium absorption, and defective bone mineralization (rickets/osteomalacia).

Clinical Manifestations

- Rickets Symptoms: Soft, weak bones leading to bowed legs or knock-knees, often evident in children as they begin walking.
- Bone Pain and Weakness: Affected individuals experience pain, especially in the lower limbs, and general muscle weakness.
- Short Stature: Delayed growth and shorter-than-average height are common, due to impaired bone growth plates.
- Dental Issues: Dental abscesses, delayed tooth eruption, enlarged pulp chambers, and weakened enamel are frequently observed.
- Hypophosphatemia: Low phosphate levels in the blood, which leads to poor bone mineralization.
- Others: Craniosynostosis in infants and sensorineural hearing loss in adults.

Genetic Diagnosis

- Routine blood tests show persistently low serum phosphate levels, elevated alkaline phosphatase levels, elevated FGF23 levels, and normal to low 1,25-dihydroxyvitamin D levels.
- Genetic Testing of the PHEX Gene: Confirmatory diagnosis is achieved by identifying pathogenic mutations in the PHEX gene through DNA sequencing and deletion/duplication analysis by MLPA. This provides definitive information for affected individuals, helps in classifying the disorder, and is crucial for cascade testing for family members at risk.

Genetic Counselling

- **Review of Medical and Family History**

  Collect a detailed three-generation family history along with consanguinity information focusing on early bone deformities, growth issues, bone pain, dental problems, and any signs suggestive of rickets or osteomalacia in relatives. This helps establish the inheritance pattern and identify at-risk individuals.

- **Discussion of Diagnosis**

  Explain the genetic basis of XLH, its X-linked dominant inheritance pattern, and the primary defect in renal phosphate handling due to the PHEX gene mutation. Discuss how the constant loss of phosphate in the kidneys, mediated by high FGF23, leads to weakened bones and characteristic rickets features. Differentiate XLH from nutritional rickets clearly.

- **Inheritance Pattern**

  XLH follows an X-linked dominant inheritance pattern, meaning that both males and females can be affected, although symptoms are often more pronounced in males. Female carriers (affected) have a 50% chance of passing the mutation to each child regardless of sex, with affected males more likely to exhibit severe symptoms. For an affected male, all daughters are affected but sons are unaffected.

- **Pre-test Counselling**

  Discuss the benefits of genetic testing for at-risk family members, especially for those planning families, to confirm carrier status and the likelihood of passing on XLH. Obtain informed consent before genetic testing. Address potential emotional and psychological concerns related to the chronic nature of the disorder and its impact on quality of life.

- **Post-test Counselling**

  Communicate test results and explain their significance, including implications for affected or carrier status, particularly for family planning. Offer recommendations for at-risk relatives to undergo testing and educate them on the importance of early diagnosis and monitoring for symptoms.

- **Medical Management and Surveillance**

  Emphasize the importance of maintaining phosphate levels with oral phosphate supplements and active forms of vitamin D (e.g., calcitriol or alfacalcidol) to improve bone mineralization, promote growth, and manage rickets/osteomalacia symptoms. Regular monitoring of serum phosphate, calcium, alkaline phosphatase, creatinine, and kidney function is essential to ensure efficacy and prevent complications. Dental care and orthopedic interventions are also important. In severe cases, growth hormone therapy may be considered to enhance growth outcomes.

- **Reproductive and Family Planning**

  Discuss reproductive options for individuals or couples at risk. These include preimplantation genetic diagnosis (PGD) in conjunction with in vitro fertilization (IVF) to select unaffected embryos. Prenatal testing via chorionic villus sampling (CVS) or amniocentesis can be considered if parents are known carriers. Discuss options such as gamete donation or adoption.

- **Psychosocial Support**

  Provide support and resources, including connections to advocacy organizations, to assist individuals and families in coping with the emotional and physical challenges associated with XLH. Address concerns about living with a chronic condition affecting bone health, mobility, and body image.

- **Follow-Up and Referrals**

  Schedule regular follow-up appointments to assess bone health, growth, response to treatment, and overall condition management. Make referrals to a multidisciplinary team including endocrinologists, nephrologists, orthopedic surgeons, dentists, physical therapists, and geneticists for comprehensive care.

- **Documentation**

  Counselling sessions should be meticulously documented, including pedigree analysis, informed consent, genetic test reports, summary of diagnosis and management discussions, and follow-up plans. Confidentiality and secure storage of records must be maintained according to institutional policies.

References

1. Haffner, D., et al. (2025). Clinical practice recommendations for the diagnosis and management of X-linked hypophosphataemia. Nature reviews. Nephrology, 21(5), 330–354.
2. Carpenter, T. O., Imel, E. A., Holm, I. A., Jan de Beur, S. M., & Insogna, K. L. (2011). A clinician's guide to X-linked hypophosphatemia. Journal of bone and mineral research : the official journal of the American Society for Bone and Mineral Research, 26(7), 1381–1388.
3. Linglart, A., et al. (2014). Therapeutic management of hypophosphatemic rickets from infancy to adulthood. Endocrine connections, 3(1), R13–R30.
4. Levine M. A. (2020). Diagnosis and Management of Vitamin D Dependent Rickets. Frontiers in pediatrics, 8, 315.

Rett Syndrome

Introduction

- Rett syndrome is a rare, progressive neurodevelopmental disorder that primarily affects females.
- It is characterized by normal early development followed by a period of regression, leading to loss of motor and communication skills.
- The disorder involves multisystem impairment including neurological, respiratory, gastrointestinal, and orthopedic systems, often with an autistic-like presentation during the regression phase.
- Early and accurate diagnosis is critical for initiating supportive care and preparing for potential future therapeutic interventions.

Genetic Etiology

- MECP2 Gene Mutation: Rett syndrome is mainly caused by mutations in the MECP2 gene on the Xq28 chromosome, which plays a crucial role in brain development and function.
- MECP2 encodes methyl-CpG-binding protein 2 (MeCP2), a crucial transcriptional regulator essential for normal brain development and synaptic maturation.
- X-Linked Dominant Inheritance: Rett syndrome follows an X-linked dominant inheritance pattern, though it generally arises from de novo mutations (90%) rather than being inherited.

- Impact on Males: Because males only have one X chromosome, they are usually more severely affected and may not survive infancy if they inherit the MECP2 mutation.

Clinical Manifestations

- Developmental Regression: After a period of typical development (6-18 months), affected individuals experience loss of motor and cognitive skills, known as developmental regression.
- Loss of Hand Skills: Rett syndrome is characterized by repetitive hand movements, such as wringing or clapping, and loss of purposeful hand use.
- Speech Impairment: Most individuals with Rett syndrome lose the ability to speak.
- Autistic Features: Symptoms may include social withdrawal, loss of eye contact, and irritability, resembling autism spectrum disorder.
- Motor Abnormalities: Includes gait abnormalities, ataxia, and muscle rigidity.
- Breathing Irregularities: These can include hyperventilation, breath-holding, and apnea.
- Seizures: Seizure disorders are common in individuals with Rett syndrome.
- Scoliosis: Progressive scoliosis often develops in late childhood or adolescence.

Genetic Diagnosis

- MECP2 Gene Testing: Genetic testing, typically by sequencing or deletion/duplication analysis, is essential to confirm MECP2 mutations.
- Differential Diagnosis: Given overlapping symptoms with other neurodevelopmental disorders, comprehensive genetic testing and clinical assessment are recommended.

- Prenatal Testing: If an MECP2 mutation is identified in a family, prenatal testing may be available to assess future pregnancies, although Rett syndrome is rarely inherited.

Genetic Counselling

- **Review of Medical and Family History**

  A detailed three-generation pedigree should be taken, including any instances of developmental delay, unexplained neurological conditions, or early childhood death. Consanguinity should be noted. As most cases are de novo, family history may be negative, but maternal mosaicism should be considered.

- **Discussion of Diagnosis**

  The diagnosis should be explained as a result of a pathogenic MECP2 mutation leading to dysregulation of neuronal gene expression. The phenotype involves severe developmental regression, with preserved eye gaze being a distinctive feature. The progressive and multisystemic nature of the disorder should be emphasized.

- **Inheritance Pattern and Recurrence Risk**

  Rett syndrome follows an X-linked dominant pattern. Nearly all cases are due to de novo mutations, particularly in paternal germline due to more frequent cell divisions during spermatogenesis. In rare familial cases, the mother may be an asymptomatic carrier (due to skewed X-inactivation). Male fetuses with MECP2 mutations usually do not survive to term or present with a more severe neonatal encephalopathy.

- **Pre-test Counselling**

  Prior to genetic testing, the family should be informed about the implications of identifying a MECP2 mutation, including diagnosis confirmation and reproductive implications. Informed consent must be obtained, and the possibility that a negative result does not excluding Rett syndrome (clinical diagnosis remains valid) should be discussed.

- **Post-test Counselling**

  Test results should be conveyed clearly, explaining whether the mutation is pathogenic, likely pathogenic, or of uncertain significance. The recurrence risk is generally low but increases if maternal mosaicism is detected. Cascade testing may be advised for the mother and other female relatives.

- **Medical Management and Surveillance**

  Management is symptomatic and requires a multidisciplinary team. Interventions include physical, occupational, and speech therapy. Monitoring for seizures, scoliosis, gastrointestinal symptoms, and nutritional needs is essential. Regular assessments by neurology, cardiology, gastroenterology, and orthopedics are recommended.

- **Reproductive and Family Planning**

  The risk of recurrence in future pregnancies is typically <1% but can increase if the mother is a carrier or mosaic. Options include prenatal testing (CVS/amniocentesis) if the familial mutation is known, and preimplantation genetic diagnosis (PGD) through IVF. Genetic counselling may include discussions of alternatives such as donor gametes or adoption, if applicable.

- **Psychosocial Support**

  Parents and caregivers often experience emotional distress. Counselling should include resources for peer support groups. Psychological support for coping with long-term care needs and the progressive nature of the disorder is essential.

- **Follow-Up and Referrals**

  Routine follow-up should include scheduled visits to neurologists, geneticists, therapists, and orthopedists. Educational specialists and social workers should be engaged for school-based support and assistive services. Coordination of care is vital for optimal outcomes.

- **Documentation**

  Comprehensive records should include the genetic counselling summary, pedigree, consent forms, test reports, management plans, and referrals. All information should be securely stored with confidentiality maintained.

References

1. Neul, J. L., et al. (2014). Developmental delay in Rett syndrome: data from the natural history study. Journal of neurodevelopmental disorders, 6(1), 20.
2. Kyle, S. M., Vashi, N., & Justice, M. J. (2018). Rett syndrome: a neurological disorder with metabolic components. Open biology, 8(2), 170216.
3. Fu, C., Armstrong, D., Marsh, E., Lieberman, D., Motil, K., et al. (2020). Consensus guidelines on managing Rett syndrome across the lifespan. BMJ paediatrics open, 4(1), e000717.
4. Noruzinia, M., Akbari, M. T., Ghofrani, M., & Sheikhha, H. (2007). Rett syndrome molecular diagnosis and implications in genetic counseling. Indian journal of human genetics, 13(3), 119–121.

CHROMOSOMAL DISORDERS

Down Syndrome

Introduction

- Down syndrome (DS), also known as trisomy 21, is the most common chromosomal cause of intellectual disability.
- It results from an extra copy of chromosome 21 and affects multiple organ systems.
- Incidence is approximately 1 in 700 live births worldwide.
- Risk increases with advanced maternal age, though most cases occur in younger women due to higher birth rates.

Genetic Etiology

- Caused by an extra copy of chromosome 21 material.
- Standard Trisomy 21 (95%): Nondisjunction during meiosis leads to three separate copies of chromosome 21 in all cells.
- Robertsonian Translocation (3–4%): Additional chromosome 21 material is attached to another chromosome, usually chromosome 14 or 21.
- Mosaicism (1–2%): Presence of two cell lines—one with normal chromosomes and one with trisomy 21—due to post-zygotic nondisjunction.

Clinical Manifestation

- Facial Features: Flat facial profile, upslanting palpebral fissures, epicanthal folds, small ears, and a flat nasal bridge.
- Neurological: Intellectual disability (mild to moderate), delayed milestones, hypotonia.
- Musculoskeletal: Joint hyperflexibility, short stature, simian crease.
- Cardiac: Congenital heart defects (about 50%), most commonly atrioventricular septal defects.
- Gastrointestinal: Duodenal atresia, Hirschsprung disease.
- Hematologic: Increased risk of leukemia, especially acute megakaryoblastic leukemia.
- Endocrine: Hypothyroidism (congenital or acquired).
- Vision and Hearing: Refractive errors, cataracts, strabismus; sensorineural or conductive hearing loss.
- Immunologic: Increased susceptibility to infections and autoimmune conditions.

Genetic Diagnosis

- Prenatal Screening:
    - First trimester combined screening: Nuchal translucency (increased thickness), PAPP-A (decreased), and β-hCG (increased).
    - Second trimester triple/quadruple screening: AFP (decreased), β-hCG (increased), estriol (decreased), inhibin A (increased).
    - Non-Invasive Prenatal Testing (NIPT): Cell-free fetal DNA testing from maternal blood (high sensitivity and specificity for trisomy 21).
- Confirmatory Testing:
    - Chorionic Villus Sampling (CVS) or Amniocentesis for fetal karyotyping.

- Postnatal Testing:
  - Karyotyping: To confirm trisomy 21 and identify type (full, mosaic, or translocation).
  - FISH (Fluorescence in situ Hybridization): Rapid aneuploidy detection for chromosome 21.
  - Chromosomal Microarray (CMA): For detecting subtle chromosomal abnormalities, although standard karyotype is sufficient for classical DS.

Genetic Counselling

- **Review of Medical and Family History**

  Obtain a comprehensive three-generation pedigree, noting any history of intellectual disability, birth defects, chromosomal anomalies, or previous children with Down syndrome. Consanguinity status should also be assessed. Family members with reproductive losses or infertility should be explored, especially in translocation-related DS.

- **Discussion of Diagnosis**

  Explain the clinical features of DS and relate them to the chromosomal findings. It is essential to link observable symptoms such as developmental delays and characteristic facial features with the underlying genetic etiology. Differences between standard trisomy, mosaic, and translocation forms should be discussed, as well as their impact on prognosis and recurrence risk.

- **Inheritance Pattern and Recurrence Risk**

  Standard trisomy 21 and mosaicism are sporadic and arise de novo due to nondisjunction. Translocation DS may be inherited and poses a significant recurrence risk, especially if a parent is a balanced translocation carrier. In such cases, karyotyping of both parents is important. The recurrence risk varies: <1% for de novo trisomy 21, 10–15% with parental translocation 13;21, 14;21, 15;21 and 100% if 21;21 translocation.

- **Pre-test Counselling**

  Before genetic testing, counsellors must explain the purpose, potential outcomes, limitations, and psychological implications of testing. Informed consent should be obtained, and counselling should cover the implications of test results for the individual and their family. For prenatal settings, the decision to test should be patient-centered and non-directive.

- **Post-test Counselling**

  Results should be communicated clearly. A confirmed diagnosis of DS should be accompanied by discussions of prognosis, medical needs, and support systems. In cases of translocation, cascade testing should be offered to at-risk family members. Counsellors should address emotional responses and offer continued psychological support.

- **Medical Management and Surveillance**

  Early intervention programs with physical, speech, and occupational therapies are essential. Regular surveillance for associated medical conditions including echocardiograms, thyroid function tests, vision and hearing evaluations are important. Immunizations and preventive care should be strictly followed. Management is best approached through a multidisciplinary team including pediatricians, cardiologists, and endocrinologists.

- **Reproductive and Family Planning**

  For families with a translocation form of DS, reproductive options include preimplantation genetic diagnosis (PGD) with IVF to select unaffected embryos, prenatal testing (by amniocentesis or CVS) in future pregnancies, and the use of donor gametes or adoption.

- **Psychosocial Support**

  Parents and families may experience a range of emotional responses. Counsellors should provide empathetic support, address grief or anxiety, and normalize adaptive strategies. Referral to local or national

Down syndrome support groups and connection with other families with shared experiences are essential.

- **Follow-Up and Referrals**

  Continued follow-up for medical surveillance, developmental evaluation, and emotional support is essential. Appropriate referrals include cardiology, endocrinology, audiology, pediatrics, and genetic services. Regular reassessment ensures timely intervention and supports long-term quality of life.

- **Documentation**

  Detailed documentation of the counselling session, informed consent for testing, pedigree analysis, and test results should be securely stored in the patient's medical record. Counsellors should ensure that all communication, risk assessments, and recommendations are recorded and secured systematically.

References

1. Antonarakis, S. E., Skotko, B. G., Rafii, M. S., Strydom, A., Pape, S. E., Bianchi, D. W., Sherman, S. L., & Reeves, R. H. (2020). Down syndrome. Nature Reviews Disease Primers, 6(1), 9.
2. Bull, M. J., & the Committee on Genetics. (2022). Health supervision for children with Down syndrome. Pediatrics, 149(5), e2022057010.
3. Sherman SL et al. Epidemiology of Down syndrome. Ment Retard Dev Disabil Res Rev. 2007;13(3):221–227.
4. Santoro, S. L., Jacobson, T., Lemle, S., & Bartman, T. (2017). Integrating a Geneticist in a Multidisciplinary Clinic for Down Syndrome Increases Commitment to Genetic Counseling. Pediatric quality & safety, 2(5), e039.

Turner Syndrome

Introduction

- Turner syndrome (TS) is a chromosomal disorder affecting females, characterized by partial or complete absence of one X chromosome (45,X).
- It has an estimated prevalence of 1 in 2,000 to 2,500 live female births.
- Clinical features include short stature, gonadal dysgenesis, and various systemic abnormalities, especially cardiac and renal anomalies.
- Early diagnosis and coordinated care are essential to optimize outcomes in affected individuals.

Genetic Etiology

- Turner syndrome results from:
  - Complete monosomy X (45,X): Most common karyotype (about 50% of cases).
  - Mosaicism (e.g., 45,X/46,XX or 45,X/46,XY): Found in about 30% of cases.
  - Structural abnormalities of the X chromosome: e.g., isochromosomes, deletions, ring chromosomes.
- The condition is typically sporadic and not inherited. It usually arises due to nondisjunction during meiosis or mitosis.

Clinical Manifestation

- Growth and skeletal features: Short stature, delayed growth, broad chest with widely spaced nipples, cubitus valgus.
- Gonadal dysgenesis: Streak ovaries leading to primary amenorrhea and infertility.
- Facial and neck features: Low posterior hairline, webbed neck, micrognathia.
- Cardiovascular anomalies: Bicuspid aortic valve, coarctation of the aorta, hypertension.
- Renal anomalies: Horseshoe kidney, duplication of the collecting system.
- Endocrine issues: Hypothyroidism, glucose intolerance.
- Neurocognitive profile: Normal intelligence, but difficulties in visuospatial skills, executive function, and nonverbal learning.
- Hearing loss and recurrent otitis media are also common.

Genetic Diagnosis

- Karyotyping: Primary method to detect monosomy X and structural abnormalities.
- FISH (Fluorescence In Situ Hybridization): Useful to detect mosaicism and low-level Y chromosome material.
- Chromosomal Microarray (CMA): Detects deletions and duplications, particularly in mosaic cases.
- Prenatal Diagnosis: By amniocentesis or chorionic villus sampling (CVS) if nuchal translucency or cystic hygroma is observed in first-trimester screening.

Genetic Counselling

- **Review of Medical and Family History**

  A comprehensive review should include a three-generation pedigree, with attention to consanguinity and recurrent pregnancy losses. Though Turner syndrome is not typically inherited, documenting family history helps rule out other X-linked or chromosomal disorders. History of infertility, delayed puberty, short stature, or congenital heart defects in female relatives should be recorded.

- **Discussion of Diagnosis**

  Explain that Turner syndrome results from a missing or structurally abnormal X chromosome and emphasize that this condition affects only females. The diagnosis should be linked to the clinical features observed such as short stature, delayed puberty, and cardiac anomalies highlighting that the genetic findings are consistent with the clinical presentation.

- **Inheritance Pattern and Recurrence Risk**

  Turner syndrome is typically sporadic and does not follow classical Mendelian inheritance. It results from nondisjunction during gametogenesis (meiosis) or early embryonic development. Recurrence risk is low, but prenatal testing may be offered in subsequent pregnancies based on family history or parental anxiety.

- **Pre-test Counselling**

  Pre-test counselling should include an explanation of the indications for genetic testing, such as clinical suspicion of Turner syndrome or abnormal prenatal ultrasound findings. The counsellor must obtain informed consent, detailing the potential outcomes and limitations of testing, including incidental findings such as low-level mosaicism or Y chromosome.

- **Post-test Counselling**

  Upon confirming the diagnosis, results must be communicated clearly. Families should be educated on the spectrum of clinical features and individualised prognosis based on the karyotype. Cascade testing for relatives is not typically necessary, but counselling should include psychological support and a plan for multidisciplinary management.

- **Medical Management and Surveillance**

  Management of Turner syndrome requires early and continuous care. Growth hormone therapy should be initiated in early childhood to optimize adult height. Estrogen replacement is necessary for pubertal induction and maintenance of secondary sexual characteristics, typically starting around 11–12 years of age. Regular cardiac screening using echocardiography or MRI is critical due to risks such as coarctation of the aorta and aortic dissection. Renal anomalies should be evaluated with ultrasound. Hearing should be monitored through periodic audiometry, and thyroid function should be screened routinely to detect autoimmune thyroiditis. Lifelong follow-up with endocrinologists, cardiologists, and gynecologists is essential to manage hormonal, cardiovascular, and reproductive health.

- **Reproductive and Family Planning**

  While infertility is common due to gonadal dysgenesis, spontaneous menarche and pregnancy may occur in individuals with mosaicism. Preconception counselling is important to evaluate cardiovascular risks before attempting pregnancy. Options such as oocyte or embryo donation with IVF, surrogacy, and adoption should be discussed. PGD is rarely indicated but may be considered in certain mosaic cases. The decision to pursue pregnancy should involve a multidisciplinary team to assess maternal risks and guide safe planning.

- **Psychosocial Support**

  Turner syndrome can affect self-esteem, social relationships, and mental health, especially due to short stature, infertility, and learning differences. Genetic counselling should include discussion of these challenges and referral to appropriate psychological support when needed. Individuals often benefit from connecting with support groups, and may require educational assistance due to nonverbal learning difficulties or attention deficits.

- **Follow-Up and Referrals**

  Ongoing care should include regular endocrinology visits for growth and hormone therapy, cardiology follow-up for structural or acquired heart disease, and gynecological support for reproductive health. Referrals to audiologists, psychologists, and special education professionals should be made as needed based on individual assessments. A coordinated multidisciplinary approach ensures timely intervention and supports optimal quality of life.

- **Documentation**

  Comprehensive documentation should include the three-generation pedigree, clinical findings, informed consent for testing, and a summary of counselling provided. Records must include diagnosis, prognosis, management plans, referrals, and follow-up recommendations. All documentation should be stored securely, respecting confidentiality and ensuring accessibility for future care.

References

1. Bondy, C. A. (2007). Care of girls and women with Turner syndrome: a guideline of the Turner Syndrome Study Group. *The Journal of Clinical Endocrinology & Metabolism*, 92(1), 10–25.
2. Sybert, V. P., & McCauley, E. (2004). Turner's syndrome. *New England Journal of Medicine*, 351(12), 1227–1238.
3. Gravholt, C. H., Viuff, M. H., Brun, S., Stochholm, K., & Andersen, N. H. (2019). Turner syndrome: mechanisms and management. Nature reviews. Endocrinology, 15(10), 601–614.

4. Villarreal, E. M. L., Prado, S. C., Schack, A. K., Sánchez, S. Á., Casado, M. A., Krych, L., & Garrido-Navas, M. C. (2025). The importance of genetic counselling for turner syndrome transition. European child & adolescent psychiatry, 34(3), 943–958.

Klinefelter Syndrome

Introduction

- Klinefelter syndrome (KS) is a common sex chromosome aneuploidy affecting males.
- It is characterized by the presence of one or more extra X chromosomes, most commonly 47,XXY.
- The condition is often underdiagnosed due to variable clinical presentation.
- It can impact physical, cognitive, and reproductive development.

Genetic Etiology

- Caused by nondisjunction during meiosis, resulting in an extra X chromosome.
- Most commonly 47,XXY karyotype; variants include 48,XXXY or 49,XXXXY.
- In 90% of cases, the extra X chromosome is of maternal origin.
- Mosaicism (46,XY/47,XXY) accounts for approximately 10% of cases and may lead to milder symptoms.

Clinical Manifestation

- Tall stature with long limbs and eunuchoid body proportions.
- Small testes, hypogonadism, gynecomastia, and infertility.

- Learning disabilities, especially in language and executive function.
- Delayed puberty, decreased facial and body hair, and low libido.
- Social difficulties and mild motor coordination problems in some individuals.

Genetic Diagnosis

- Karyotyping: Standard method for confirming 47,XXY or mosaic variants.
- FISH: Useful for detecting low-level mosaicism.
- Chromosomal microarray (CMA): May incidentally detect KS during prenatal or pediatric genetic testing.
- Hormonal testing: Elevated FSH and LH, low testosterone levels.

Genetic Counselling

- **Review of Medical and Family History**

  A comprehensive three-generation pedigree should be taken to evaluate any familial patterns of developmental delays, infertility, or chromosomal abnormalities. Although Klinefelter syndrome is typically sporadic, it is essential to record consanguinity, previous reproductive history, or recurrent pregnancy loss.

- **Discussion of Diagnosis**

  The counsellor should explain that KS is a chromosomal condition involving an extra X chromosome in males, leading to the characteristic clinical features. The diagnosis is typically made via chromosomal analysis (karyotyping). Symptoms like infertility, small testes, and delayed puberty align with the genetic findings, reinforcing the diagnosis.

- **Inheritance Pattern and Recurrence Risk**

  KS is not inherited in a Mendelian pattern but occurs due to random chromosomal nondisjunction. Recurrence risk in families is low, and no carrier testing is needed. In some cases, mosaicism (e.g., 46,XY/47,XXY) may occur, leading to variable phenotypic expression, often with milder clinical features and a higher chance of preserved fertility.

- **Pre-test Counselling**

  Pre-test counselling should emphasize the purpose of genetic testing, especially in individuals with infertility, gynecomastia, or developmental concerns. Informed consent must be obtained, highlighting possible incidental findings and implications for reproductive health.

- **Post-test Counselling**

  Results should be conveyed with clarity, including explanations of standard vs. mosaic karyotypes. For individuals diagnosed postnatally, counselling should cover implications for fertility, hormonal health, and psychosocial support. Family members may be offered counselling, although cascade testing is not usually required.

- **Medical Management and Surveillance**

  Early endocrinologic intervention is essential. Testosterone replacement therapy is indicated in most cases, typically initiated at puberty. Regular evaluations by endocrinologists and psychologists are recommended. Monitor for osteoporosis, metabolic syndrome, and breast cancer risk.

- **Reproductive and Family Planning**

  Most individuals with KS are infertile due to azoospermia, but assisted reproductive techniques such as testicular sperm extraction (TESE) combined with intracytoplasmic sperm injection (ICSI) may offer biological parenthood in selected cases. Options like sperm donation or adoption should be discussed. Genetic counselling is critical in preconception planning.

- **Psychosocial Support**

  Supportive counselling is essential to address emotional and psychological aspects related to delayed diagnosis, infertility, or body image issues. Involvement in patient advocacy groups and support networks can improve self-esteem and adherence to therapy. Educational assistance may be needed for language-based learning difficulties.

- **Follow-Up and Referrals**

  Regular follow-up with an endocrinologist is essential for hormonal monitoring. Referrals should include speech therapists, psychologists, and urologists. A multidisciplinary approach ensures optimal outcomes across the lifespan.

- **Documentation**

  Detailed notes should be maintained, including informed consent for testing, test results, interpretation, counselling session summaries, management plans, and referrals made. All records must be securely stored in compliance with medical confidentiality standards.

References

1. Lanfranco, F., Kamischke, A., Zitzmann, M., & Nieschlag, E. (2004). Klinefelter's syndrome. The Lancet, 364(9430), 273-283.
2. Groth, K. A., Skakkebæk, A., Høst, C., Gravholt, C. H., & Bojesen, A. (2013). Clinical review: Klinefelter syndrome--a clinical update. The Journal of clinical endocrinology and metabolism, 98(1), 20–30.
3. Skakkebaek, A., Wallentin, M., & Gravholt, C. H. (2015). Neuropsychology and socioeconomic aspects of Klinefelter syndrome: new developments. Current opinion in endocrinology, diabetes, and obesity, 22(3), 209–216.
4. Herlihy, A. S., et al. (2011). Diagnosis and management of Klinefelter syndrome: An Australian perspective. The Medical Journal of Australia, 194(9), 552-556.

DiGeorge Syndrome

Introduction

- DiGeorge syndrome (DGS), also known as 22q11.2 deletion syndrome, is a common microdeletion syndrome characterized by a spectrum of clinical features including congenital heart defects, immunodeficiency, palatal anomalies, hypocalcemia, and developmental delay.
- It results from a deletion in chromosome 22 at the q11.2 region and affects approximately 1 in 4,000 live births.
- Clinical presentation is variable, ranging from mild to life-threatening manifestations.
- Early diagnosis is crucial for timely medical management and developmental support.

Genetic Etiology

- Caused by a hemizygous deletion of a 1.5 to 3 Mb segment on chromosome 22q11.2.
- The deletion affects approximately 30–40 genes, notably the TBX1 gene, which is critical for the development of the pharyngeal system.
- Most cases are de novo (about 90%), but autosomal dominant inheritance is possible in familial cases.
- Parental chromosomal testing is essential to determine recurrence risk.

Clinical Manifestation

- Cardiac anomalies: Conotruncal defects like tetralogy of Fallot, interrupted aortic arch, ventricular septal defects.
- Immunodeficiency: Due to thymic hypoplasia or aplasia, leading to T-cell deficiency.
- Hypocalcemia: Resulting from hypoparathyroidism, especially in the neonatal period.
- Palatal abnormalities: Cleft palate, velopharyngeal insufficiency, hypernasal speech.
- Facial features: Mild dysmorphic features including hooded eyelids, small chin, and prominent nasal root.
- Neurodevelopmental and psychiatric issues: Delayed speech/language, learning disabilities, ADHD, and increased risk for schizophrenia in adolescence or adulthood.
- Other anomalies: Renal malformations, hearing loss, skeletal anomalies.

Genetic Diagnosis

- Fluorescence in situ hybridization (FISH) using probes specific for the 22q11.2 region is a conventional method.
- Multiplex ligation-dependent probe amplification (MLPA) is a reliable, cost-effective technique for detecting deletions.
- Chromosomal microarray (CMA) is the gold standard for diagnosis, allowing detection of submicroscopic deletions and differentiating overlapping syndromes.
- Quantitative PCR and next-generation sequencing (NGS)-based CNV analysis are also used.
- Parental testing is recommended when a child is diagnosed with 22q11.2 deletion to determine whether the deletion is inherited.

Genetic Counselling

- **Review of Medical and Family History**

  A detailed three-generation pedigree should be obtained, with attention to congenital heart disease, immunodeficiency, speech delay, cleft palate, psychiatric disorders, or unexplained neonatal deaths. Consanguinity should also be documented, although DGS is typically not associated with consanguineous inheritance.

- **Discussion of Diagnosis**

  The diagnosis of DGS is based on clinical findings consistent with the syndrome and confirmed by molecular cytogenetic testing. Genetic counselling should explain the spectrum of features due to the 22q11.2 deletion and clarify the variable expressivity, even within families.

- **Inheritance Pattern and Recurrence Risk**

  DGS follows an autosomal dominant pattern. While most cases are de novo, approximately 10% are inherited from an affected parent. If a parent carries the deletion, the recurrence risk for offspring is 50%. De novo cases carry a low recurrence risk, but parental testing is essential to confirm the origin.

- **Pre-test Counselling**

  Pre-test counselling should address the purpose of genetic testing, potential findings, implications for the individual and family, and psychological impact. Informed consent must be obtained before testing, and reproductive implications should be discussed for reproductive-age individuals or couples.

- **Post-test Counselling**

  Test results should be explained in detail. In confirmed cases, cascade testing for parents and siblings should be offered. Negative results may not rule out DGS if clinical suspicion remains, in which case higher-resolution techniques for diagnosis may be considered. Implications for other family members should be clearly communicated.

- **Medical Management and Surveillance**

  Management is multidisciplinary and should begin early. This includes cardiology evaluation and surgical intervention as required, calcium monitoring and supplementation, immune evaluation, vaccination, and hearing assessments. Growth, nutrition, speech, and developmental progress must be regularly monitored. Neurodevelopmental assessment and psychiatric support are important.

- **Reproductive and Family Planning**

  Counselling for affected individuals should address the autosomal dominant inheritance and 50% recurrence risk. Options such as preimplantation genetic diagnosis (PGD) or prenatal testing via chorionic villus sampling (CVS) or amniocentesis should be offered. Donor gametes or adoption may be discussed when appropriate.

- **Psychosocial Support**

  Families should be supported in dealing with the chronic and multifaceted nature of the condition. Referral to national or regional support groups and mental health professionals is recommended. Additional resources for special school-based support should be discussed.

- **Follow-Up and Referrals**

  Lifelong follow-up is essential. Referrals should be made to cardiologists, immunologists, endocrinologists, ENT specialists, speech and occupational therapists, pediatricians, and psychiatrists. Periodic multidisciplinary evaluations helps to anticipate and manage complications.

- **Documentation**

  All counselling sessions, informed consent forms, diagnostic reports, family history details, and management plans should be meticulously recorded. Secure and confidential storage of genetic information is mandatory, especially for future reproductive planning.

References

1. McDonald-McGinn, D. M., Sullivan, K. E., Marino, B., Philip, N., Swillen, A., Vorstman, J. A., Zackai, E. H., Emanuel, B. S., Vermeesch, J. R., Morrow, B. E., Scambler, P. J., & Bassett, A. S. (2015). 22q11.2 deletion syndrome. Nature reviews. Disease primers, 1, 15071.
2. McDonald-McGinn, D. M., & Zackai, E. H. (2008). Genetic counseling for the 22q11.2 deletion. Developmental disabilities research reviews, 14(1), 69–74.
3. Bassett AS, et al. Practical guidelines for managing patients with 22q11.2 deletion syndrome. J Pediatr. 2011;159(2):332-339.e1.

DEVELOPMENTAL DISORDERS

Developmental Delay

Introduction

- Developmental delay refers to a significant lag in a child's physical, cognitive, behavioural, emotional, or social development compared to normative age milestones.
- It may be global (affecting multiple domains) or specific (e.g., speech or motor skills alone).
- Genetic causes are increasingly recognized as significant contributors, particularly when delays are unexplained by environmental or perinatal factors.

Genetic Etiology

- Chromosomal abnormalities (e.g., Down syndrome, Fragile X syndrome, microdeletions).
- Single-gene disorders (e.g., Rett syndrome, tuberous sclerosis, metabolic disorders).
- Copy number variations (CNVs) and pathogenic mutations identified through chromosomal microarray or exome sequencing.
- Mitochondrial disorders or imprinting disorders.
- Multifactorial causes involving both genetic and environmental factors.

Clinical Manifestation

- Delayed milestones in speech/language, gross or fine motor skills, cognition, or social interaction.
- Hypotonia or hypertonia.
- Dysmorphic facial features.
- Seizures, vision or hearing impairments.
- Behavioural features (e.g., autism spectrum traits, hyperactivity).
- Associated physical anomalies (e.g., cardiac or renal malformations).

Genetic Diagnosis

- Clinical assessment: Detailed developmental and medical history, family history, physical and neurological examination.
- Chromosomal Microarray Analysis (CMA): First-tier test for unexplained developmental delay/intellectual disability.
- Fragile X Testing: Recommended for all boys with unexplained developmental delay.
- Whole Exome Sequencing (WES) or targeted gene panels: Useful when initial testing is negative.
- Metabolic screening: Indicated if clinical signs suggest an inborn error of metabolism.
- Neuroimaging (MRI): May be required if neurological findings or structural anomalies are present.

Genetic Counselling

- **Review of Medical and Family History**

  Draw a detailed three-generation pedigree to identify inheritance patterns, consanguinity, history of developmental delay, intellectual disability, miscarriages, or congenital anomalies in the family.

Medical records review, prenatal and perinatal histories, and early developmental assessments are also essential.

- **Discussion of Diagnosis**

  Counsellors explain the concept of developmental delay, emphasizing that genetic causes may be contributing factors, especially in the absence of environmental impact. Clinical findings should be correlated with known genetic syndromes, if applicable. The explanation should be individualised based on the suspected or confirmed diagnosis, using simple language to ensure family understanding.

- **Inheritance Pattern and Recurrent Risk**

  Inheritance patterns vary based on the underlying genetic cause; autosomal dominant, autosomal recessive, X-linked, de novo, or mitochondrial. Mosaicism and variable expressivity may account for differences in phenotype among relatives with the same genetic condition. If no clear inheritance pattern is observed, de novo mutation or multifactorial causes are considered.

- **Pre-test Counselling**

  Families are counselled on the purpose, scope, and limitations of genetic testing. Informed consent must be obtained after explaining test accuracy, possible outcomes (diagnostic, uncertain, or negative), implications for management, and reproductive risks. The potential need for additional testing based on results is discussed.

- **Post-test Counselling**

  Counsellors provide detailed interpretations of test results and their clinical significance. A pathogenic finding may allow for targeted management, recurrence risk assessment, and cascade testing in relatives. Uncertain results (variants of uncertain significance) should be explained carefully. Negative results do not exclude a genetic basis and may require re-evaluation or further advanced testing.

- **Medical Management and Surveillance**

  Management depends on the underlying diagnosis but commonly includes early intervention services such as physiotherapy, speech therapy, and occupational therapy. Multidisciplinary follow-up is essential for managing associated medical issues. Regular developmental assessments help in planning educational and therapeutic interventions.

- **Reproductive and Family Planning**

  Counselling includes recurrence risk assessment for future pregnancies and available reproductive options such as preimplantation genetic diagnosis (PGD), prenatal testing (CVS, amniocentesis), or gamete donation. Families with known genetic diagnoses benefit from precise risk estimates and planning.

- **Psychosocial Support**

  The diagnosis of developmental delay can be emotionally overwhelming. Counsellors must address parental guilt, stress, or anxiety. Referral to local or regional support groups and connecting with other families with similar experiences can aid in coping. Educational materials and resources should be provided.

- **Follow-Up and Referrals**

  Follow-up includes re-evaluation after genetic test results, monitoring developmental progress, and periodic updates on evolving medical issues. Referrals are made to neurologists, pediatricians, clinical geneticists, physical, speech, and occupational therapies, and special-school education professionals as needed.

- **Documentation**

  A complete record of the counselling session should include the clinical summary, family pedigree, informed consent, details of the genetic test offered, interpretation of results, and follow-up plan. All documents must be securely stored, maintaining confidentiality.

References

1. Moeschler, J. B., Shevell, M., & Committee on Genetics (2014). Comprehensive evaluation of the child with intellectual disability or global developmental delays. Pediatrics, 134(3), e903–e918.
2. Miller, D. T., et al. (2010). Consensus statement: chromosomal microarray is a first-tier clinical diagnostic test for individuals with developmental disabilities or congenital anomalies. American journal of human genetics, 86(5), 749–764.
3. Srour, M., & Shevell, M. (2014). Genetics and the investigation of developmental delay/intellectual disability. Archives of disease in childhood, 99(4), 386–389.
4. Savatt, J. M., & Myers, S. M. (2021). Genetic Testing in Neurodevelopmental Disorders. Frontiers in pediatrics, 9, 526779.

Neurodevelopmental Disorders

Introduction

- Neurodevelopmental disorders (NDDs) encompass a group of conditions characterized by impairments in cognitive, motor, language, and social development.
- Common examples include global developmental delay (GDD), intellectual disability (ID), autism spectrum disorder (ASD), and attention-deficit hyperactivity disorder (ADHD).
- NDDs can result from genetic, environmental, or multifactorial causes, with genetic factors being a significant contributor.

Genetic Etiology

- Genetic causes include:
  - Chromosomal abnormalities (e.g., Down syndrome, 22q11.2 deletion)
  - Single-gene disorders (e.g., Rett syndrome, Fragile X syndrome)
  - Copy number variants (CNVs)
  - Mitochondrial disorders and inborn errors of metabolism
- In many cases, the genetic etiology may be complex or remain undiagnosed despite testing.

Clinical Manifestation

- Delay in achieving developmental milestones (motor, speech, social).
- Intellectual disability, ranging from mild to severe.
- Behavioural concerns such as hyperactivity, autism traits, or aggression.
- Associated comorbidities like seizures, hypotonia, dysmorphic features, or feeding difficulties.
- Some children may show regression of previously acquired skills.

Genetic Diagnosis

- Chromosomal Microarray (CMA): First-line test to detect microdeletions or duplications (CNVs).
- Fragile X testing: Especially in males with ID or autism traits.
- Whole Exome Sequencing (WES): Recommended if CMA and Fragile X are non-diagnostic.
- Targeted gene panels: Depending on clinical suspicion (e.g., ASD, epilepsy).
- Metabolic screening: If clinical features suggest a metabolic disorder.
- Karyotyping: For suspected aneuploidies or balanced rearrangements.

Genetic Counselling

- **Review of Medical and Family History**

  A thorough three-generation pedigree should be obtained, noting any relatives with similar developmental issues, intellectual disability, seizures, or unexplained infant deaths. Parental consanguinity should be recorded, especially in populations where consanguineous marriages are common, as this increases the likelihood of autosomal recessive disorders.

- **Discussion of Diagnosis**

  Explain that neurodevelopmental disorders are heterogeneous in cause and presentation. While some diagnoses are evident based on clinical and genetic testing, others remain elusive. It is important to correlate developmental delays and associated features with the likely or confirmed genetic etiology and to clarify that testing may or may not yield a definitive result.

- **Inheritance Pattern and Recurrence Risk**

  The inheritance pattern depends on the underlying diagnosis. Chromosomal abnormalities: Usually de novo but may be inherited (e.g., translocations). Single-gene disorders: May follow autosomal dominant, autosomal recessive, or X-linked patterns. CNVs: Often de novo but can be inherited, particularly if involving susceptibility loci. Mosaicism or variable penetrance may lead to phenotypic variability even within families.

- **Pre-test Counselling**

  Genetic testing should be performed after obtaining informed consent, with discussion on possible outcomes (positive, negative, variant of uncertain significance), turnaround time, cost, and limitations of testing. Parents should be made aware that testing may impact family members and may have reproductive implications.

- **Post-test Counselling**

  Results should be communicated clearly, including the clinical significance and any incidental findings. If a pathogenic variant is identified, cascade testing for at-risk relatives should be offered. If no diagnosis is found, this should be explained as part of the diagnostic limitations and not as an exclusion of a genetic cause.

- **Medical Management and Surveillance**

  Management of neurodevelopmental disorders is multidisciplinary, involving coordinated care from pediatricians, neurologists, psychologists, and allied health professionals such as speech and occupational therapists. Early intervention services play a crucial role in supporting developmental milestones. Regular surveillance is necessary to identify and address comorbidities including epilepsy, visual or hearing impairments, and behavioural challenges. Nutritional and feeding issues should also be assessed and managed through appropriate referrals.

- **Reproductive and Family Planning**

  Parents should be counselled regarding the recurrence risk of the child's neurodevelopmental condition, based on the confirmed or suspected inheritance pattern. Genetic options such as carrier screening (particularly for autosomal recessive and X-linked conditions), prenatal testing via chorionic villus sampling or amniocentesis, and preimplantation genetic diagnosis (PGD) through IVF should be discussed. For couples at high risk of recurrence, the use of donor gametes or adoption may also be considered.

- **Psychosocial Support**

  Psychological support for the family is essential to address grief, anxiety, and expectations. Referral to parent support groups, special school education resources, and community-based services can help parents feel less isolated and better equipped to manage the child's condition.

- **Follow-Up and Referrals**

  Regular follow-up with the genetic counsellor is essential for updated testing recommendations and support. Referrals should include pediatricians, neurologists, physical, speech, and occupational therapists, and special school educators. Families may also need access to social workers and mental health professionals.

- **Documentation**

  Records should include a detailed three-generation pedigree, clinical notes, informed consent forms, and all genetic test requisitions and results. Counselling summaries should include key discussion points, risk assessments, and follow-up recommendations. All documents must be stored securely with appropriate confidentiality and restricted access.

References

1. Morris-Rosendahl, D. J., & Crocq, M. A. (2020). Neurodevelopmental disorders-the history and future of a diagnostic concept . Dialogues in clinical neuroscience, 22(1), 65–72.
2. Thapar, A., Cooper, M., & Rutter, M. (2017). Neurodevelopmental disorders. The lancet. Psychiatry, 4(4), 339–346.
3. Rossi, M., El-Khechen, D., Black, M. H., Farwell Hagman, K. D., Tang, S., & Powis, Z. (2017). Outcomes of Diagnostic Exome Sequencing in Patients With Diagnosed or Suspected Autism Spectrum Disorders. Pediatric neurology, 70, 34–43.e2.
4. Blesson, A., & Cohen, J. S. (2020). Genetic Counseling in Neurodevelopmental Disorders. Cold Spring Harbor perspectives in medicine, 10(4), a036533.

Dysmorphic Child

Introduction

- A dysmorphic child presents with congenital anomalies and/or distinct physical features that deviate from typical development and morphology.
- Dysmorphic features may suggest an underlying genetic syndrome, chromosomal abnormality, or teratogenic exposure.
- Early evaluation is crucial for diagnosis, management, and family counselling.

Genetic Etiology

- Dysmorphology can result from chromosomal abnormalities (e.g., trisomy 21, microdeletions), single-gene disorders (e.g., Noonan syndrome), or multifactorial causes.
- De novo mutations, inherited syndromes, or environmental exposures during embryogenesis may contribute.
- Disruptions in developmental pathways affecting organogenesis and morphogenesis are common mechanisms.

Clinical Manifestation

- Craniofacial anomalies: hypertelorism, epicanthal folds, micrognathia, low-set ears.

- Skeletal anomalies: clinodactyly, limb length discrepancies, syndactyly.
- Growth abnormalities: short stature, microcephaly or macrocephaly.
- Neurological signs: developmental delay, hypotonia, seizures.
- Organ malformations: cardiac defects, renal anomalies, gastrointestinal atresia.
- Skin findings: café-au-lait spots, hypopigmentation, unusual hair distribution.

Genetic Diagnosis

- Detailed clinical evaluation and dysmorphology assessment by a clinical geneticist or trained clinician.
- Chromosomal Microarray (CMA): First-tier test for unexplained dysmorphism and developmental delay; detects copy number variants.
- Karyotyping: Useful in detecting aneuploidy (e.g., Down syndrome, Turner syndrome) or balanced rearrangements.
- Targeted gene panels or exome sequencing: Used when a monogenic disorder is suspected.
- Metabolic workup: If inborn errors of metabolism are suspected based on clinical presentation.

Genetic Counselling

- **Review of Medical and Family History**

  A thorough review of medical records and clinical presentation is essential, with a focus on birth history, prenatal exposures, and developmental milestones. A three-generation pedigree should be constructed to identify patterns of inheritance and consanguinity. Details of previous miscarriages, stillbirths, and known genetic conditions in the family should be documented.

- **Discussion of Diagnosis**

  The diagnosis may remain uncertain in many dysmorphic children; hence, the counsellor must explain that the evaluation is often stepwise. When features are consistent with a known syndrome, the relationship between phenotype and genotype should be outlined. When a molecular diagnosis is confirmed, its implications for prognosis and management should be discussed clearly with the family.

- **Inheritance Pattern and Recurrence Risk**

  The inheritance pattern varies depending on the underlying cause: autosomal dominant (e.g., Noonan syndrome), autosomal recessive (e.g., Ellis-van Creveld syndrome), X-linked (e.g., Aarskog syndrome), or chromosomal. In many cases, especially those due to de novo mutations or chromosomal anomalies, recurrence risk is low but not zero due to possible gonadal mosaicism.

- **Pre-test Counselling**

  Genetic testing should be preceded by detailed pre-test counselling explaining the purpose, types of tests recommended, potential outcomes (positive, negative, variants of uncertain significance), limitations, and implications for management and family members. Informed consent must be obtained and documented.

- **Post-test Counselling**

  Results should be communicated clearly. If a diagnosis is confirmed, cascade testing should be offered to relevant family members. If results are inconclusive, further evaluation or periodic reanalysis may be discussed. Counselling should include information on recurrence risk and the need for reproductive counselling.

- **Medical Management and Surveillance**

  Multidisciplinary management, involving clinical geneticists, pediatricians, physical, speech, and occupational therapies, cardiologists, neurologists, and other subspecialists depending on associated anomalies. Surveillance is guided by syndrome-specific protocols, focusing on early detection and management of complications.

- **Reproductive and Family Planning**

  Parents should be offered recurrence risk assessment based on the identified etiology and parental genetic testing results. Options include prenatal testing (CVS/amniocentesis), preimplantation genetic diagnosis (PGD), and gamete donation. Counselling should address the emotional, ethical, and medical implications of each choice.

- **Psychosocial Support**

  Parents may experience anxiety, guilt, or distress. Counsellors should provide empathetic support and connect families with syndrome-specific foundations, early intervention programs, and family support groups. Psychological counselling may be beneficial for coping and adjustment.

- **Follow-Up and Referrals**

  Follow-up should be scheduled for continued counselling, coordination of care, and psychosocial support. Referrals may include paediatrics, physical, speech, and occupational therapies, audiology, cardiology, ophthalmology, and support networks.

- **Documentation**

  Comprehensive documentation must include the pedigree, clinical findings, informed consent, genetic test reports, counselling notes, management plan, and follow-up recommendations. Records must be stored securely in accordance with confidentiality standards.

References

1. Wright, C. F., FitzPatrick, D. R., & Firth, H. V. (2018). Paediatric genomics: diagnosing rare disease in children. Nature reviews. Genetics, 19(5), 253–268.
2. Ciancia, S., Madeo, S. F., Calabrese, O., & Iughetti, L. (2024). The Approach to a Child with Dysmorphic Features: What the Pediatrician Should Know. Children (Basel, Switzerland), 11(5), 578.
3. Biesecker, L. G., Adam, M. P., Alkuraya, F. S., Amemiya, A. R., Bamshad, M. J., et al. (2021). A dyadic approach to the delineation of diagnostic entities in clinical genomics. American journal of human genetics, 108(1), 8–15.
4. Kaufman, J., & White, S. M. (2017). An approach to the child with dysmorphic features. Journal of paediatrics and child health, 53(3), 221–222.
5. Levkova, M., Stoyanova, M., Hachmeriyan, M. et al (2024). A cost-efficient algorithm for diagnosing children with dysmorphic features. Egypt J Med Hum Genet 25, 76.

Ambiguous Genitalia

Introduction

- Ambiguous genitalia refers to external genitalia that do not have the typical appearance of either a male or female infant.
- It is a medical emergency and requires immediate evaluation to determine underlying etiology and appropriate gender assignment.
- It is a feature of disorders/differences of sex development (DSDs), which include a spectrum of congenital conditions.

Genetic Etiology

- May result from chromosomal abnormalities (e.g., 45,X/46,XY mosaicism), single-gene disorders, or enzymatic defects.
- Congenital adrenal hyperplasia (CAH) due to 21-hydroxylase deficiency (autosomal recessive) is the most common cause in genetic females (46,XX).
- Androgen insensitivity syndrome (X-linked) is a common cause in 46,XY individuals.
- Mutations in genes such as SRD5A2, NR5A1, and SRY may lead to under-virilization or gonadal dysgenesis.

Clinical Manifestation

- Atypical genitalia at birth (e.g., enlarged clitoris, micropenis, fused labia, hypospadias).
- Palpable gonads may indicate the presence of testicular tissue.
- Salt-wasting crisis in CAH (vomiting, dehydration, hypotension).
- Absent or atypical internal reproductive structures.
- Family history of consanguinity or similar conditions may be present.

Genetic Diagnosis

- Karyotyping to determine chromosomal sex and detect large structural abnormalities.
- Chromosomal microarray (CMA) to detect copy number variations
- FISH for locating SRY gene in individuals with 46,XX or 46,XY DSD.
- Targeted molecular testing based on phenotype (e.g., CYP21A2 for CAH, AR gene for androgen insensitivity, SRD5A2 for 5-alpha reductase deficiency).
- Hormonal assays: 17-hydroxyprogesterone, testosterone, DHEAS, LH/FSH, cortisol, electrolytes, and AMH (anti-Mullerian hormone).
- Imaging (pelvic ultrasound or MRI) to assess internal genitalia and gonads.

Genetic Counselling

- **Review of Medical and Family History**

  A three-generation pedigree should be obtained, documenting any history of genital ambiguity, infertility, early neonatal deaths (suggestive of adrenal crisis), pubertal abnormalities, or consanguinity. Review prenatal history, perinatal course, and previous genetic or hormonal test results if available.

- **Discussion of Diagnosis**

  The counsellor should explain the differential diagnosis for ambiguous genitalia, linking observed physical features and hormone levels with possible underlying genetic or enzymatic defects. It is important to discuss the urgency of identifying potentially life-threatening causes (e.g., salt-wasting CAH) and the immediate and long-term implications for gender assignment, medical management, psychosocial well-being, and potential future fertility.

- **Inheritance Pattern and Recurrent Risk**

  The inheritance pattern in cases of ambiguous genitalia varies depending on the underlying etiology. Congenital adrenal hyperplasia (CAH) caused by mutations in the CYP21A2 gene and 5-alpha-reductase deficiency (SRD5A2), follow an autosomal recessive inheritance. X-linked inheritance is observed in disorders like complete and partial androgen insensitivity syndrome, where mutations affect the AR gene. In some cases, such as gonadal dysgenesis or NR5A1-related disorders of sex development (DSDs), mutations may occur de novo or may be inherited in either autosomal dominant or recessive patterns, depending on the specific gene and mutation. Counsellors should clearly outline recurrence risks for future pregnancies based on the identified cause.

- **Pre-test Counselling**

  Pre-test counselling involves explaining the purpose and implications of karyotyping, molecular, and hormonal tests. Parents should be informed about the need for urgent testing in certain cases, the possible results, and how they may influence gender assignment and management. Informed consent should be obtained, including discussions on privacy, potential incidental findings, and psychological impact of a DSD diagnosis.

- **Post-test Counselling**

  Test results must be communicated sensitively and clearly, including an explanation of the underlying diagnosis and implications for medical and gender management. When a genetic cause is identified, cascade testing may be recommended for at-risk relatives. Discuss the possible need for gender reassignment or confirmatory interventions in light of new findings. Provide accurate, age-appropriate information as the child grows.

- **Medical Management and Surveillance**

  Management requires a multidisciplinary team, including endocrinologists, urologists, surgeons, and psychologists. Medical therapy may include hormone replacement, surgical correction, and monitoring for adrenal crisis in CAH. Lifelong follow-up is necessary to address growth, pubertal development, fertility, and psychosocial adaptation.

- **Reproductive and Family Planning**

  Once the diagnosis is confirmed, parents should be counselled on recurrence risks and available options. These include carrier screening, prenatal testing via chorionic villus sampling or amniocentesis, and preimplantation genetic diagnosis (PGD) for future pregnancies. For the child, future reproductive potential depends on the etiology and gonadal function.

- **Psychosocial Support**

  Families may experience distress, confusion, grief, isolation, and anxiety. It is essential to provide psychosocial counselling to help them cope with the diagnosis, gender identity decisions, and societal attitudes. Referral to specialized DSD support groups and families with shared experience is encouraged. Long-term psychological support for the individual with DSD should be advised.

- **Follow-Up and Referrals**

  Regular follow-up should be arranged with a multidisciplinary DSD team. Referrals may include endocrinology, pediatric urology/surgery, clinical genetics, and child psychology/psychiatry. Educational interventions may be needed based on developmental assessments.

- **Documentation**

  Thorough documentation is important. It should include the pedigree, detailed physical examination findings, informed consent for testing, test results, counselling session summaries, gender assignment decisions, and long-term management plans. Records should be maintained with strict confidentiality and handled with sensitivity, respecting the individual's evolving understanding of their sex development.

References

1. Yatsenko, S. A., & Witchel, S. F. (2017). Genetic approach to ambiguous genitalia and disorders of sex development: What clinicians need to know. Seminars in perinatology, 41(4), 232–243.
2. Ahmed, S. F., Bashamboo, A., Lucas-Herald, A., & McElreavey, K. (2013). Understanding the genetic aetiology in patients with XY DSD. British medical bulletin, 106, 67–89.
3. Lee, P. A., et al & Global DSD Update Consortium (2016). Global Disorders of Sex Development Update since 2006: Perceptions, Approach and Care. Hormone research in paediatrics, 85(3), 158–180.
4. Amor, D. (2020). Genetic counselling. In J. Hutson, S. Grover, M. O'Connell, A. Bouty, & C. Hanna (Eds.), Disorders/differences of sex development (pp. 279-292). Springer.

REPRODUCTIVE GENETICS

Recurrent Pregnancy Loss

Introduction

- Recurrent pregnancy loss (RPL) is defined as the occurrence of two or more consecutive pregnancy losses before 20 weeks of gestation.
- Affects approximately 1–2% of couples trying to conceive.
- Causes may be genetic, anatomical, hormonal, autoimmune, infectious, thrombophilic, endocrine, environmental or unexplained.
- Genetic evaluation plays a crucial role in identifying underlying causes and guiding future reproductive options.

Genetic Etiology

- Chromosomal abnormalities account for 2–5% of RPL cases.
- The most common genetic cause is balanced chromosomal rearrangement (e.g., reciprocal or Robertsonian translocations or inversions) in one of the parents.
- Aneuploidies (e.g., trisomy, monosomy, polyploidy) in the embryo, often due to maternal age-related meiotic errors, are a major cause of sporadic miscarriage but can contribute to RPL.
- Single gene disorders and copy number variations (CNVs) may be implicated in some cases, especially with fetal anomalies.

Clinical Manifestation

- History of two or more spontaneous miscarriages, typically before 20 weeks.
- May or may not be associated with fetal anomalies identified on ultrasound or postmortem examination.
- Couples may report infertility, grief, emotional distress, and increased anxiety with future pregnancies.

Genetic Diagnosis

- Parental karyotyping: This is a standard first-tier test to detect balanced translocations or inversions in either parent.
- Product of conception (POC) testing: Chromosomal microarray (CMA) or karyotype of fetal tissue to identify aneuploidies or CNVs. CMA can detect CNVs that karyotyping might not detect.
- Next-generation sequencing panels: Offered in selected cases for identifying monogenic causes or recurrent fetal anomalies. Whole exome sequencing (WES) may be considered in complex, undiagnosed cases.
- Prenatal testing: In subsequent pregnancies if a genetic abnormality is identified.
- Preimplantation genetic testing: PGT-SR may be advised in cases with parental chromosomal rearrangements or PGT-A, or couples with a history of recurrent aneuploidy, especially with advanced maternal age.

Genetic Counselling

- **Review of Medical and Family History**

  A comprehensive three-generation pedigree should be obtained, documenting previous miscarriages, stillbirths, or neonatal deaths, consanguinity, and any family history of congenital anomalies or known genetic conditions. Reproductive history including gestational age at loss, ultrasound findings, or autopsy reports of prior pregnancies should be carefully reviewed.

- **Discussion of Diagnosis**

  Counsellors should explain the potential genetic basis for RPL, emphasizing that while some causes are identifiable, others may remain unexplained despite testing. If a parental chromosomal rearrangement or genetic anomaly is found, its contribution to pregnancy loss should be explained in relation to the clinical history and findings, including the mechanism by which it leads to non-viable pregnancies.

- **Inheritance Pattern and Recurrence Risk**

  In couples with a balanced translocation, the pattern is usually autosomal dominant with a risk of producing unbalanced gametes, leading to miscarriage or offspring with congenital anomalies and/or intellectual disability. The empirical risk for liveborn unbalanced offspring varies significantly by the specific translocation. Fetal aneuploidies may be sporadic but their incidence significantly increases with advanced maternal age. In rarer cases, autosomal recessive, X-linked, or de novo single gene mutations may contribute to RPL, especially if there are recurrent fetal anomalies or specific syndromic presentations. Accurate risk estimation depends critically on the specific genetic finding.

- **Pre-test Counselling**

  Genetic testing should be preceded by informed consent, explaining the purpose, benefits, limitations, and possible outcomes. Discuss implications for future pregnancies, emotional impact of results, and possible need for further reproductive decision-making based on outcomes. Address potential incidental findings, cost implications, and turnaround time for results

- **Post-test Counselling**

  Test results should be interpreted and communicated clearly. If a parental chromosomal rearrangement is detected, cascade testing may be offered to other family members who may also be balanced carriers. For couples with a history of aneuploidies or CNVs, recurrence risks and options such as preimplantation testing or early prenatal diagnosis should be discussed.

- **Medical Management and Surveillance**

  Management may include referral to endocrinology for assisted reproduction options or to maternal-fetal medicine for high-risk pregnancy care. Early ultrasonography and close antenatal surveillance may be needed in subsequent pregnancies. Address associated medical conditions such as thrombophilia, diabetes, or thyroid dysfunction, as these can be independent causes of RPL.

- **Reproductive and Family Planning**

  Couples with recurrent pregnancy loss should be informed of reproductive options based on the underlying genetic findings. Preimplantation genetic testing (PGT) with IVF enables selection of unaffected embryos in cases of known chromosomal or monogenic disorders. Prenatal diagnosis via chorionic villus sampling (CVS) or amniocentesis may be offered in future pregnancies. Donor gametes or adoption should be discussed when genetic risks are high. Counselling must support informed, value-aligned decisions.

- **Psychosocial Support**

  Couples experiencing RPL often face profound grief, anxiety, and depression. Genetic counselling should offer empathetic emotional support and facilitate referral to mental health professionals. Support groups, both local and regional, can provide valuable connection with others experiencing similar losses.

- **Follow-Up and Referrals**

  Structured follow-up is essential to review results, provide ongoing emotional support, and guide future reproductive planning. Couples may be referred to a clinical geneticist for further evaluation and a fertility specialist for assisted conception options. Maternal-fetal medicine consultation is important in high-risk pregnancies. Psychologists and social workers may assist with emotional and logistical support. Continued access to counselling enhances patient outcomes.

- **Documentation**

  Each counselling session must be thoroughly documented, including a three-generation pedigree and detailed reproductive history. Notes should include informed consent, test requisitions, and key discussion points on risks and options. Summaries must include the diagnosis, genetic implications, and agreed follow-up plan. All documents should be stored securely, ensuring strict confidentiality and accessibility only to authorized personnel.

References

1. Melo, P., Dhillon-Smith, R., Islam, M. A., Devall, A., & Coomarasamy, A. (2023). Genetic causes of sporadic and recurrent miscarriage. Fertility and sterility, 120(5), 940-944.
2. Practice Committee of the American Society for Reproductive Medicine (2012). Evaluation and treatment of recurrent pregnancy loss: a committee opinion. Fertility and sterility, 98(5), 1103–1111.
3. van den Berg, M. M., van Maarle, M. C., van Wely, M., & Goddijn, M. (2012). Genetics of early miscarriage. Biochimica et biophysica acta, 1822(12), 1951–1959.
4. Hyde, K. J., & Schust, D. J. (2015). Genetic considerations in recurrent pregnancy loss. Cold Spring Harbor perspectives in medicine, 5(3), a023119.

Infertility

Introduction

- Infertility is defined as the inability to conceive after 12 months of regular, unprotected intercourse.
- It affects approximately 10–15% of couples worldwide and may be due to male, female, combined, or unexplained factors.
- Genetic causes are implicated in 15–30% of infertility cases, especially when standard clinical and laboratory workups are inconclusive.
- Genetic counselling plays a vital role in identifying hereditary contributions, assessing recurrence risk, and guiding reproductive options.

Genetic Etiology

- Male factors: Common causes include Klinefelter syndrome (47,XXY), Y-chromosome microdeletions (AZF regions), CFTR mutations associated with congenital bilateral absence of vas deferens (CBAVD), and chromosomal translocations.
- Female factors: Premature ovarian insufficiency (POI), Turner syndrome (45,X or mosaics), Fragile X premutation (FMR1), and mutations in genes such as BMP15 and FOXL2.
- Combined/Unknown: Mutations in genes affecting gametogenesis, fertilization, and early embryonic development.

Clinical Manifestation

- Male infertility: Azoospermia, oligospermia, abnormal sperm morphology or motility, delayed puberty, small testes, or gynecomastia.
- Female infertility: Amenorrhea, oligomenorrhea, short stature, primary ovarian insufficiency, or absence of secondary sexual characteristics.
- Family history: Reproductive anomalies, early menopause, infertility, or consanguinity may be present.
- Associated features: May include dysmorphic features, developmental delay, or endocrine disorders.

Genetic Diagnosis

- Karyotyping: Used to identify aneuploidies (e.g., 47,XXY) and structural chromosomal abnormalities (e.g., balanced translocations, inversions) in either partner.
- Y-Chromosome Microdeletion Analysis: A standard test in males with non-obstructive azoospermia or severe oligospermia; performed via PCR to detect deletions in the AZFa, AZFb, and AZFc regions.
- CFTR Gene Testing: Indicated in males with CBAVD to assess risk of cystic fibrosis in offspring, especially if the female partner is also a *CFTR* carrier.
- FMR1 Testing: Recommended in women with premature ovarian insufficiency or family history of Fragile X-related disorders.
- Targeted gene panels: May be used in idiopathic infertility via NGS-based multigene panels, depending on clinical suspicion.
- Whole Exome Sequencing (WES) may be considered in complex, undiagnosed cases, particularly with syndromic features.
- Hormonal assays: Essential for clinical diagnosis and guiding genetic testing, including FSH, LH, estradiol, testosterone, and AMH (Anti-Müllerian Hormone).

Genetic Counselling

- **Review of Medical and Family History**

  A thorough evaluation includes personal medical history (including childhood development, puberty, surgeries, chronic illnesses, and relevant medication use), consanguinity, menstrual or pubertal abnormalities, and previous ART attempts. A three-generation pedigree helps identify inherited conditions, chromosomal anomalies, or patterns suggestive of X-linked or autosomal conditions contributing to infertility and to identify other affected or carrier relatives.

- **Discussion of Diagnosis**

  The diagnosis should be explained in the context of reproductive history and clinical findings. For example, a man with azoospermia and a Yq microdeletion should be counselled on the genetic basis, the lack of natural fertility, the need for assisted reproduction, and the implications for male offspring. For females, findings like FMR1 premutation or Turner syndrome should be linked with premature ovarian failure/infertility risk, associated health risks, and potential for mosaicism.

- **Inheritance Pattern and Recurrence Risk**

  Inheritance patterns vary based on the underlying disorder. Klinefelter syndrome and Turner syndrome typically result from de novo aneuploidy, leading to a very low recurrence risk for future pregnancies. Y-chromosome microdeletions follow a paternal inheritance if passed (affected males transmit to all sons), while CFTR mutations and other monogenic causes follow autosomal recessive or dominant patterns. X-linked patterns may be noted in FMR1-related cases. Counsellors must clarify recurrence risks, discussing the potential for de novo mutations and inherited forms.

- **Pre-test Counselling**

  Counsellors must discuss the purpose and scope of genetic testing, including karyotyping, microdeletion analysis, and gene sequencing. Informed consent is mandatory, particularly in contexts like ART, where genetic results may influence reproductive decision-making (e.g., choice of donor gametes, use of PGT). Emotional preparedness, psychosocial implications, and potential for incidental findings or variants of uncertain significance (VUS) should also be discussed.

- **Post-test Counselling**

  Test results should be interpreted in a supportive and informative manner. Positive findings may affect family members (e.g., CFTR mutation carrier status, balanced chromosomal rearrangement) and necessitate cascade testing. Negative or inconclusive results should be contextualized, emphasizing limitations of current genetic technology and potential for future reanalysis as new genes or diagnostic methods emerge. Discuss the option of revisit if new information on a VUS becomes available.

- **Medical Management and Surveillance**

  Management includes ART options like IVF, ICSI (intracytoplasmic sperm injection), and surgical sperm or oocyte retrieval. Individuals with Klinefelter syndrome or POI may require hormonal therapy. Men with Yq microdeletion may be candidates for surgical sperm extraction, but the risk of transmission to all male offspring and resulting infertility in them should be addressed. Ongoing medical support and surveillance depend on the underlying diagnosis and associated health risks.

- **Reproductive and Family Planning**

  Counselling should support informed choices aligned with the couple's values, preferences, and personal goals. Reproductive options for couples with genetic causes of infertility include:

    - IVF with ICSI, often used when sperm count is very low or sperm require surgical extraction.
    - Preimplantation genetic testing (PGT) (including PGT-A for aneuploidy, PGT-SR for structural rearrangements, and PGT-M for monogenic conditions) may be advised in couples with known chromosomal or monogenic conditions to reduce the risk of affected offspring or implantation failure.
    - Prenatal diagnosis via CVS or amniocentesis may be relevant where significant genetic risks exist for offspring (e.g., balanced translocations, carrier parents)
    - Donor gametes or adoption in couples with significant genetic risks, failed ART attempts, or when biological parenthood is not possible or desired.

- **Psychosocial Support**

  Infertility can have profound emotional, psychological, and social effects, including grief, anxiety, depression, guilt, and marital strain. Counsellors should address these psychological distresses, the stigma often associated with infertility, and expectations from family or society. Referral to fertility counsellors, support groups, and peer networks can be instrumental in providing coping strategies and a sense of community. Acknowledging cultural sensitivities and offering non-directive counselling promotes autonomy and informed decision-making.

- **Follow-Up and Referrals**

  Follow-up is essential to provide continued support, track reproductive decisions, and manage evolving clinical or genetic findings. Referral may include endocrinologists, urologists, fertility clinics, geneticists, psychologists, and social workers. Genetic follow-up may be required if additional testing (e.g., re-evaluation of VUS) or cascade testing for relatives is recommended.

- **Documentation**

  All sessions should be documented thoroughly, including pedigree charts, consent forms, testing recommendations, results, and detailed reproductive counselling discussions. Confidentiality should be strictly maintained, and medical records securely stored for future reference, especially in cases with ART interventions or hereditary implications for extended family.

References

1. Practice Committee of the American Society for Reproductive Medicine. Electronic address: asrm@asrm.org, & Practice Committee of the American Society for Reproductive Medicine (2021). Fertility evaluation of infertile women: a committee opinion. Fertility and sterility, 116(5), 1255–1265.
2. Practice Committee of the American Society for Reproductive Medicine (2015). Diagnostic evaluation of the infertile male: a committee opinion. Fertility and sterility, 103(3), e18–e25.
3. Yatsenko, S. A., & Rajkovic, A. (2019). Genetics of human female infertility†. Biology of reproduction, 101(3), 549–566.
4. Krausz, C., & Riera-Escamilla, A. (2018). Genetics of male infertility. Nature reviews. Urology, 15(6), 369–384.
5. Liker, K., Black, L., Weil, J., Bruce, J., Bereknyei Merrell, S., Bivona, S., & Ormond, K. E. (2019). Challenges of infertility genetic counseling: Impact on counselors' personal and professional lives. Journal of genetic counseling, 28(3), 626–640.

Carrier Screening in Couples

Introduction

- Carrier screening identifies individuals or couples who carry gene mutations that may cause autosomal recessive or X-linked conditions in their offspring.
- It is typically offered preconceptionally or in early pregnancy to facilitate informed reproductive decision-making.
- Carrier screening may be population-specific/targeted (based on ethnicity/family history) or expanded (covering multiple genes irrespective of background).
- Early identification allows for risk assessment, reproductive planning, and timely intervention.

Genetic Etiology

- Autosomal recessive conditions require both partners to be carriers of mutations in the same gene (e.g., thalassemia, cystic fibrosis).
- X-linked conditions involve mutations in genes on the X chromosome, where female carriers can pass the disorder to male offspring (e.g., Duchenne muscular dystrophy)
- Pathogenic variants in these genes may not cause symptoms in carriers but can significantly affect offspring if inherited in combination.

Clinical Manifestation

- Carrier individuals are typically asymptomatic.
- If both partners are carriers, offspring may be at risk for:
    - Autosomal recessive conditions: 25% affected, 50% carriers, 25% unaffected.
    - X-linked conditions: 50% of sons affected if the mother is a carrier; 50% daughters may be carriers.
- Disorders screened vary in severity and age of onset; many are serious, life-limiting, or disabling.

Genetic Diagnosis

- Targeted testing is based on known familial mutations or ethnic-specific conditions.
- Expanded carrier screening (ECS) panels assess for >100 genes regardless of ancestry.
- Molecular techniques used include next-generation sequencing (NGS), multiplex PCR, and deletion/duplication analysis.
- Results should specify the mutation, zygosity, and residual risk where applicable.

Genetic Counselling

- **Review of Medical and Family History**

  A thorough family history, including consanguinity and known genetic disorders in the extended family, is essential. A three-generation pedigree helps identify at-risk individuals and guide appropriate test selection.
- **Discussion of Diagnosis**

  Counsellors must explain that being a carrier does not mean the individual is affected but may pass on a genetic mutation to children.

The severity, treatment options, and long-term outcomes of the conditions identified in screening must be described in understandable and non-technical terms.

- **Inheritance Pattern and Recurrence Risk**

  The inheritance pattern (autosomal recessive, X-linked, or rarely autosomal dominant with reduced penetrance) is critical in accurately estimating recurrence risk for offspring. Couples in which both partners are carriers for the same autosomal recessive condition face a 25% recurrence risk with each pregnancy. X-linked inheritance poses a 50% risk to male offspring from carrier mothers, with daughters having a 50% chance of being carriers.

- **Pre-test Counselling**

  Before testing, informed consent must be obtained, discussing the scope of the testing methodology, potential outcomes (positive/negative/variant of uncertain significance), implications for reproductive planning, and the possibility of residual risk even after negative results.

- **Post-test Counselling**

  Post-test sessions should clearly explain test results, especially if both partners are carriers of the same gene or if X-linked risk is identified. For positive results, discuss the specific genetic condition, its clinical features, prognosis, and management options. For negative results, explain the residual risk and the limitations of the screening. For VUS results, explain that these are often inconclusive and may not impact current reproductive decisions unless further studies clarify their pathogenicity. Cascade testing may be advised for family members. Discussing emotional responses and ensuring understanding of reproductive options is important.

- **Medical Management and Surveillance**

  Though carriers typically require no medical intervention, identification of carrier status may prompt partner testing, family screening, and reproductive decision-making. For high-risk couples, early prenatal diagnostic options should be advised with appropriate obstetric care.

- **Reproductive and Family Planning**

  For couples identified as being at increased risk, discuss the reproductive options. Natural conception with prenatal diagnosis (Chorionic villus sampling/amniocentesis) to determine the genetic status of the fetus. In vitro fertilization (IVF) with preimplantation genetic testing for monogenic conditions (PGT-M) to select embryos that are unaffected by the condition. Use of donor gametes, or adoption. Counselling must support decisions in accordance with personal values, beliefs, and resources.

- **Psychosocial Support**

  Discovering carrier status, particularly if both partners are carriers or an X-linked risk is identified, may lead to significant anxiety, guilt, or relationship strain. Provide reassurance, empathetic support, and access to psychosocial resources, peer support networks, or advocacy organizations specific to the condition(s) of concern. Support should empower the couples to make decisions aligned with their personal preferences.

- **Follow-Up and Referrals**

  Couples with identified risks should be referred to reproductive specialists, clinical geneticists, and maternal-fetal medicine experts. Regular follow-up ensures continuity of care and addresses evolving questions or reproductive decisions.

- **Documentation**

  Detailed records should include pedigree, test consent, laboratory reports, discussion notes, and reproductive plans. Confidential storage with controlled access is essential to ensure privacy and continuity of care.

References

1. Henneman L, et al. (2016). Responsible implementation of expanded carrier screening. European journal of human genetics : EJHG, 24(6), e1–e12.
2. Edwards JG, et al. (2015).Expanded carrier screening in reproductive medicine—points to consider. *Obstet Gynecol.* 2015;125(3):653–662.
3. Grody, W. W., Thompson, B. H., Gregg, A. R., Bean, L. H., Monaghan, K. G., Schneider, A., & Lebo, R. V. (2013). ACMG position statement on prenatal/preconception expanded carrier screening. Genetics in medicine : official journal of the American College of Medical Genetics, 15(6), 482–483.
4. Sagaser, K. G., Malinowski, J., Westerfield, L., Proffitt, J., Hicks, M. A., Toler, T. L., Blakemore, K. J., Stevens, B. K., & Oakes, L. M. (2023). Expanded carrier screening for reproductive risk assessment: An evidence-based practice guideline from the National Society of Genetic Counselors. Journal of genetic counseling, 32(3), 540–557.
5. Edwards, S., & Laing, N. (2022). Genetic Counselling Needs for Reproductive Genetic Carrier Screening: A Scoping Review. Journal of personalized medicine, 12(10), 1699.

CANCER GENETICS

Familial adenomatous polyposis

Introduction

- Familial Adenomatous Polyposis (FAP) is an inherited cancer predisposition syndrome.
- It is characterized by the development of hundreds to thousands of colorectal adenomatous polyps.
- Without timely medical intervention, nearly all affected individuals will develop colorectal cancer, often before age 40.
- It accounts for about 1% of all colorectal cancers.
- Early diagnosis and genetic counselling are key to effective management and cancer prevention.

Genetic Etiology

- Familial adenomatous polyposis (FAP) is an autosomal dominant disorder.
- It is caused by mutations in the APC (adenomatous polyposis coli) gene located on chromosome 5q21-q22.
- This gene encodes a tumor suppressor protein involved in regulating cell proliferation and division.
- Mutations in the APC gene lead to the development of numerous colorectal polyps, which have the potential to progress to colorectal cancer if left untreated.

- Attenuated FAP (AFAP) is a milder form of FAP, characterized by fewer colorectal polyps (typically <100), later onset of cancer, and variable extracolonic manifestations.

Clinical manifestations

- Colorectal Polyps - hundreds to thousands of adenomatous polyps in the colon and rectum, typically beginning in adolescence or early adulthood. These polyps increase the risk of colorectal cancer significantly.
- Extracolonic Manifestations: desmoid tumors, osteomas, dental abnormalities, congenital hypertrophy of the retinal pigment epithelium (CHRPE), and epidermoid cysts, gastric/duodenal polyps and cancer.
- Symptoms: anemia, rectal bleeding, diarrhea, abdominal pain, and changes in bowel habits due to the presence of polyps.
- Risk of Colorectal Cancer: individuals with FAP have a nearly 100% lifetime risk of developing colorectal cancer, usually by the age of 40.
- Family History: affected individuals often have a family history of the condition. However, approximately 25% of cases result from de novo mutations. Somatic mosaicism can lead to milder or segmental polyposis.

Genetic Diagnosis

- Sequencing the APC gene to identify pathogenic variants (mutations) that are associated with the condition.
- Testing includes sequencing of the entire gene or targeted analysis for specific mutations known to be associated with FAP. If a pathogenic variant is identified in the APC gene, it confirms the diagnosis of FAP.
- Deletion/duplication analysis by MLPA is sometimes used to detect large structural variants in the APC gene.

Genetic Counselling

- **Review of medical and family history**

  Gather detailed information about the affected individual's medical history, including symptoms, number of polyps, age of onset, extracolonic manifestations, other relevant diagnostic tests or procedures performed, family history of colorectal cancers or related conditions using a three-generational pedigree chart, and consanguinity information.

- **Discussion of Diagnosis**

  Explain what FAP is, how it is inherited, and its associated risks, including the development of colorectal cancer and other related conditions. How variable expressivity and incomplete penetrance can affect the severity and clinical presentation of the disorder in different individuals should be discussed. Briefly outline the concept of attenuated FAP if relevant to the family history.

- **Inheritance Pattern and Recurrence Risk**

  FAP follows an autosomal dominant inheritance pattern with high penetrance; hence, the individual has a 50% chance of inheriting the APC gene mutation from an affected parent and a 50% chance of transmitting it to each offspring. Variable expressivity may be seen within families, with differing ages of polyp development or cancer onset. The counsellor should discuss the likelihood of other family members being affected and provide information about genetic testing options for family members who may be at risk. De novo mutations occur in approximately 15-20% of cases.

- **Pre-test counselling**

  Discuss the role of genetic testing in confirming a diagnosis of FAP and determining the specific genetic mutation responsible for the condition. Outline the benefits, limitations, and implications of genetic testing, including potential psychological and emotional considerations, and facilitate informed decision-making regarding whether to proceed with genetic testing.

- **Post-test counselling**

  Communicate the genetic test results to the individual or family, providing clear explanations and answering any questions or concerns that may arise. Interpret the test results in the context of the individual's medical and family history, explaining the implications of positive, negative, or inconclusive results. If a pathogenic variant is found, at-risk family members should be offered genetic testing to identify those who carry the mutation and require early screening and management. For high-risk individuals with a negative result, explain that regular medical check-ups should continue, as some mutations might be missed by current testing techniques.

- **Medical Management and Surveillance**

  Review the recommended management and surveillance protocols for individuals with FAP and emphasize the importance of regular clinical evaluations and monitoring. Discuss the high risk of developing numerous colorectal polyps and colorectal cancer if left untreated. Explain the importance of regular colonoscopy screenings and the potential need for prophylactic surgery to prevent colorectal cancer. Address surveillance for gastric, duodenal, and other extracolonic cancers.

- **Reproductive and Family Planning**

  If applicable, the counsellor should discuss reproductive options and family planning considerations for the affected individual and other family members, including prenatal testing, preimplantation genetic diagnosis (PGD), and gamete donation or adoption.

- **Psychosocial Support**

  Diagnosis of FAP, particularly in children or adolescents, may evoke significant anxiety related to lifelong cancer risk, extensive surveillance, surgical interventions, and potential impacts on body image or fertility. Genetic counselling should include emotional support and guidance to help individuals and families cope with the challenges of living with FAP. The counsellor should address any concerns, fears, or psychosocial issues that the family may be experiencing and provide resources for additional support services, such as support groups and mental health counselling.

- **Follow-Up and Referrals**

  Schedule follow-up appointments as needed to monitor the individual's condition, provide ongoing support, and address any new questions or concerns that arise. They may also refer the family to other healthcare providers or specialists, including gastroenterologists, surgeons, geneticists, and mental health professionals, for multidisciplinary care.

- **Documentation**

  Counselling sessions must be well documented, including pedigree analysis, genetic test results, consent forms, detailed interpretation of genetic findings, discussion of management plans, and a structured follow-up plan. Storage of records must comply with confidentiality and legal standards.

References

1. Grover, S., Kastrinos, F., Steyerberg, E. W., et al. (2012). Prevalence and Phenotypes of APC and MUTYH Mutations in Patients With Multiple Colorectal Adenomas. JAMA, 308(5), 485–492.
2. Syngal, S., Brand, R. E., Church, J. M., et al. (2015). ACG Clinical Guideline: Genetic Testing and Management of Hereditary Gastrointestinal Cancer Syndromes. Am J Gastroenterol, 110(2), 223–262.
3. Kyriakidis, F., Kogias, D., Venou, T. M., Karlafti, E., & Paramythiotis, D. (2023). Updated Perspectives on the Diagnosis and Management of

Familial Adenomatous Polyposis. The application of clinical genetics, 16, 139–153.

4. Fernández-Suárez, A., Cordero Fernández, C., García Lozano, R., Pizarro, A., Garzón, M., & Núñez Roldán, A. (2005). Clinical and ethical implications of genetic counselling in familial adenomatous polyposis. Revista espanola de enfermedades digestivas, 97(9), 654–665.

Hereditary Breast and Ovarian Cancer Syndrome

Introduction

- Hereditary Breast and Ovarian Cancer (HBOC) syndrome is a genetic condition associated with a significantly increased risk of breast and ovarian cancer.
- It is most commonly linked to pathogenic variants in the *BRCA1* and *BRCA2* genes.
- HBOC accounts for approximately 5–10% of all breast cancers and 10–15% of all ovarian cancers.
- It can also be associated with other malignancies including prostate, pancreatic, and male breast cancer.

Genetic Etiology

- Caused primarily by mutations in the *BRCA1* (chromosome 17q21) and *BRCA2* (chromosome 13q13.1) tumor suppressor genes.
- Both genes are involved in DNA repair specifically homologous recombination, a high-fidelity pathway for repairing double-strand breaks.
- Inheritance is autosomal dominant with age-dependent incomplete penetrance.

- Other genes like *PALB2*, *TP53*, *CHEK2*, BRIP1 and *RAD51C/D* can also be involved in broader hereditary breast cancer syndromes.

Clinical Manifestation

- Early-onset breast cancer (<50 years).
- Triple-negative breast cancer (ER-, PR-, HER2-) is more commonly associated with BRCA1 pathogenic variants, regardless of age of onset.
- Bilateral breast cancer or multiple primary cancers in the same individual.
- High-grade serous ovarian carcinoma.
- Male breast cancer particularly with BRCA2 pathogenic variants
- Pancreatic cancer, and prostate cancer in the family or individual
- Ashkenazi Jewish ancestry with a personal or family history of breast or ovarian cancer is a significant indicator, as specific founder mutations are common in this population.

Genetic Diagnosis

- Multigene panel testing by next-generation sequencing (NGS) is the current standard.
- Testing includes full sequencing and deletion/duplication analysis of *BRCA1/2* and other high/moderate-risk genes based on personal and family history.
- Predictive testing for at-risk family members should focus on known familial mutations once identified.
- Tumor testing for BRCA mutations (especially in ovarian or triple-negative breast cancer) may guide therapeutic decisions.

Genetic Counselling

- **Review of Medical and Family History**

  Counselling begins with a detailed three-generation pedigree assessing personal and familial history of breast, ovarian, pancreatic, prostate, and related cancers (including melanoma, fallopian tube cancer, peritoneal cancer). History of early-onset, bilateral, or multiple primaries should be flagged. Consanguinity, ethnicity (e.g., Ashkenazi Jewish ancestry), and any prior genetic testing results are recorded.

- **Discussion of Diagnosis**

  Counsellors should explain the role of BRCA1/2 and related genes in DNA repair and cancer risk. Emphasize that HBOC increases the lifetime risk for specific cancers and that penetrance varies by gene, specific mutation, and gender. Provide lifetime risk estimates for various cancers associated with BRCA1 and BRCA2. The clinical presentation should be correlated with the genetic findings to guide personalized risk management strategies.

- **Inheritance Pattern and Recurrence Risk**

  HBOC is inherited in an autosomal dominant manner. Each first-degree relative of a mutation carrier has a 50% chance of inheriting the mutation. Male carriers can transmit the mutation equally to sons and daughters and are themselves at increased risk for certain cancers. Variable expressivity and age-dependent incomplete penetrance are common, meaning some carriers may never develop cancer, or may develop it at different ages, making individual risk prediction challenging.

- **Pre-test Counselling**

  Prior to genetic testing, individuals must be informed about the possible results (positive, negative, or variant of uncertain significance - VUS) and their implications for medical management and potential psychosocial impacts. Counselling should address issues of anxiety, insurability, and implications for family members. Informed consent is essential, and cascade testing should be planned if a pathogenic variant is detected.

- **Post-test Counselling**

  Results must be explained clearly and empathetically. A positive result confirms increased cancer risk and necessitates enhanced surveillance and consideration of risk-reducing strategies. A negative result in a family with a known mutation provides significant reassurance. VUS results should not influence management, but families should be informed about the possibility of reclassification. Cascade testing for at-risk relatives should be offered. Discuss the impact of the result on screening recommendations for different family members.

- **Medical Management and Surveillance**

  Management includes increased surveillance (e.g., annual MRI and mammography from age 25), chemoprevention (e.g., tamoxifen), and risk-reducing surgeries (e.g., prophylactic mastectomy and salpingo-oophorectomy). Male carriers should undergo prostate screening and have awareness of breast changes. Ovarian screening remains limited in effectiveness but is considered on a case-by-case basis. Pancreatic cancer and melanoma screening can be considered for those with strong family history.

- **Reproductive and Family Planning**

  Counselling should discuss reproductive options such as preimplantation genetic testing for monogenic conditions (PGT-M) with IVF to avoid transmission of BRCA mutations. Prenatal testing (CVS/amniocentesis) may also be considered. Reproductive decision-making should respect personal values, cultural considerations, and the complex ethical implications of testing for adult-onset conditions.

- **Psychosocial Support**

  Genetic counselling should address emotional responses to hereditary cancer risk, including anxiety, guilt, or fear. Referral to support groups and local peer networks can be helpful. Mental health support may be needed for individuals coping with diagnosis, decision-making, and long-term surveillance.

- **Follow-Up and Referrals**

  Coordinate care with a multidisciplinary team including oncologists, surgeons, gynecologists, gastroenterologists (for pancreatic risk), reproductive specialists, and psychologists/social workers as needed. Provide long-term follow-up to address emerging needs, review family updates, discuss new research and guidelines, and support ongoing decision-making regarding surveillance and interventions.

- **Documentation**

  Document informed consent, pedigree, genetic test results, and discussion details including risks, management, and referrals. Secure and confidential record-keeping is essential for future reference and family testing.

References

1. Malhotra, H., et al (2020). Genetic Counseling, Testing, and Management of HBOC in India: An Expert Consensus Document from Indian Society of Medical and Pediatric Oncology. JCO global oncology, 6, 991–1008.
2. Sessa, C., et al (2023). Risk reduction and screening of cancer in hereditary breast-ovarian cancer syndromes: ESMO Clinical Practice Guideline. Annals of oncology : official journal of the European Society for Medical Oncology, 34(1), 33–47.
3. Paluch-Shimon, S., et al. (2016). Prevention and screening in BRCA mutation carriers and other breast/ovarian hereditary cancer

syndromes: ESMO Clinical Practice Guidelines for cancer prevention and screening. Annals of oncology : official journal of the European Society for Medical Oncology, 27(suppl 5), v103–v110.

4. Agnese, D. M., & Pollock, R. E. (2016). Breast Cancer Genetic Counseling: A Surgeon's Perspective. Frontiers in surgery, 3, 4.

Lynch Syndrome

Introduction

- Lynch syndrome is the most common hereditary colorectal cancer syndrome.
- It accounts for approximately 3% of all colorectal cancer cases.
- It significantly increases the lifetime risk of various malignancies, especially colorectal and endometrial cancers.
- Early detection and surveillance significantly reduce morbidity and mortality.
- It is also known as hereditary nonpolyposis colorectal cancer (HNPCC).

Genetic Etiology

- Caused by pathogenic variants in DNA mismatch repair (MMR) genes: MLH1, MSH2, MSH6, PMS2, and deletion in EPCAM (leading to MSH2 silencing due to promoter methylation).
- These genes are responsible for correcting errors during DNA replication.
- Loss of MMR function leads to microsatellite instability (MSI) and accumulation of somatic mutations.
- Inheritance is autosomal dominant.
- Mutations are inherited from one affected parent in approximately 90% of cases.

Clinical Manifestation

- Increased lifetime risk of colorectal cancer (up to 80%), often presenting before age 50.
- Elevated risk of endometrial cancer (up to 60%), especially in females, and often presenting as the sentinel cancer.
- Other associated malignancies include ovarian, stomach, small intestine, urinary tract, pancreas, hepatobiliary tract, brain (Turcot syndrome), and skin (Muir-Torre variant).
- Tumors often show microsatellite instability (MSI-high) and/or loss of MMR protein expression on immunohistochemistry.
- Individuals typically do not present with hundreds of polyps, distinguishing it from FAP.

Genetic Diagnosis

Tumor testing

- Immunohistochemistry (IHC) for MMR proteins (MLH1, MSH2, MSH6, PMS2) in colorectal or endometrial tumors is the first-line screening step. Loss of expression of one or more proteins indicates MMR deficiency.
- Microsatellite instability (MSI) analysis (PCR-based) assesses for changes in the length of microsatellite repeats. MSI-High status indicates MMR deficiency.
- BRAF V600E mutation testing and/or MLH1 promoter methylation analysis may be performed if IHC shows isolated loss of MLH1, to differentiate sporadic from inherited MMR deficiency.

Germline testing

- Next-generation sequencing (NGS) panel to identify pathogenic variants in MLH1, MSH2, MSH6, PMS2, or EPCAM. This is performed if tumor testing suggests Lynch syndrome or if clinical criteria are met.

- EPCAM deletion testing (e.g., MLPA or other copy number analysis techniques) should be performed if MSH2 germline testing is negative but its expression is lost on IHC, or if family history strongly suggests Lynch syndrome.
- Cascade testing: Offered to first-degree relatives and other at-risk family members once the familial pathogenic variant is identified.
- Universal screening: Recommended for all newly diagnosed colorectal and endometrial cancers, regardless of age, to identify potential Lynch syndrome cases

Genetic Counselling

- **Review of Medical and Family History**

  The evaluation begins with a comprehensive three-generation pedigree focusing on colorectal, endometrial, and other Lynch-associated cancers. Information on age at diagnosis, tumor pathology reports, and history of consanguinity should be gathered. Particular attention should be paid to families meeting standard (NCCN) guidelines for Lynch syndrome genetic testing.

- **Discussion of Diagnosis**

  Genetic counsellors should explain that Lynch syndrome is due to an inherited mutation in a mismatch repair gene. The diagnosis is made based on personal and family history, tumor screening, and genetic testing. The presence of MSI or loss of MMR protein expression in tumors strongly supports the diagnosis. Emphasize that this is a manageable condition with proactive surveillance and risk-reducing strategies.

- **Inheritance Pattern and Recurrence Risk**

  Lynch syndrome follows an autosomal dominant inheritance pattern. Each first-degree relative of an affected individual has a 50% chance of inheriting the pathogenic variant. Males and females are equally affected. De novo mutations are rare but possible. Phenotypic expression may vary depending on the gene involved (e.g., MSH6 and PMS2 mutations often present later in life). The concept of incomplete penetrance should also be discussed.

- **Pre-test Counselling**

  Prior to testing, individuals must be counselled regarding the implications of identifying a hereditary cancer syndrome. Counsellors should discuss benefits, limitations, psychological impact, and potential discrimination. Informed consent should cover confidentiality, implications for insurance, and the possibility of variants of uncertain significance (VUS).

- **Post-test Counselling**

  Post-test counselling involves communicating the results, including pathogenic variants, negative results, or VUS. For positive results, cascade testing of at-risk relatives is recommended. In case of VUS, regular surveillance should continue based on personal and family history. Negative results must be interpreted in the context of family findings.

- **Medical Management and Surveillance**

  Regular colonoscopic surveillance starting from 20–25 years or 2–5 years before the earliest case in the family is crucial. Endometrial cancer surveillance may include transvaginal ultrasound and endometrial biopsy. Prophylactic hysterectomy and bilateral salpingo-oophorectomy may be considered after childbearing especially for MLH1 and MSH2 carriers due to higher ovarian cancer risks. Surveillance for upper GI and urinary tract cancers may also be indicated depending on the gene involved.

- **Reproductive and Family Planning**

  Counselling should include reproductive options such as preimplantation genetic diagnosis (PGD) for couples wishing to avoid transmission. Prenatal diagnosis may also be discussed. Carrier testing for adult children is usually deferred until age 18 or later unless early surveillance is planned.

- **Psychosocial Support**

  Patients may experience anxiety, guilt, or distress after a Lynch syndrome diagnosis. Referral to psychosocial support services and connection with support groups can be beneficial. Counselling should address the emotional impact of cancer risk and the burden of regular surveillance.

- **Follow-Up and Referrals**

  Patients should be followed regularly to ensure adherence to surveillance guidelines and to adapt recommendations as new evidence emerges. Referrals should be made to gastroenterologists, geneticists, urologists, oncologists specializing in other Lynch-associated cancers, psychologists, and cancer clinics as needed. Updates on new management recommendations or family testing options should be communicated.

- **Documentation**

  Documentation should include a detailed pedigree, test consent forms, test reports, and a summary of counselling sessions. Surveillance recommendations and referrals should be clearly outlined. Secure, confidential storage of records is essential for ongoing care and future reference.

References

1. Vasen, H. F., et al. (2013). Revised guidelines for the clinical management of Lynch syndrome (HNPCC): recommendations by a group of European experts. Gut, 62(6), 812–823.
2. Bhattacharya, P., Leslie, S. W., & McHugh, T. W. (2024). Lynch Syndrome (Hereditary Nonpolyposis Colorectal Cancer). StatPearls.

3. Kim, J. Y., & Byeon, J. S. (2019). Genetic Counseling and Surveillance Focused on Lynch Syndrome. Journal of the anus, rectum and colon, 3(2), 60–68.

4. Holter, S., et al. (2022). Risk assessment and genetic counseling for Lynch syndrome - Practice resource of the National Society of Genetic Counselors and the Collaborative Group of the Americas on Inherited Gastrointestinal Cancer. Journal of genetic counseling, 31(3), 568–583.

Retinoblastoma

Introduction

- Retinoblastoma is a rare pediatric ocular malignancy that arises from the retina.
- It typically presents in early childhood, usually before the age of five.
- It may occur in heritable (germline) or non-heritable (somatic) forms.
- Early diagnosis and management are crucial to preserve life and vision.

Genetic Etiology

- Retinoblastoma is an autosomal dominant disorder
- It is caused by mutations in the RB1 gene, which is located on chromosome 13q14. RB1 was the first tumor suppressor gene to be described.
- Loss of one RB1 allele predisposes to cancer, while loss of the second allele, in developing retinal cells, leads to retinoblastoma thereby following "two-hit model" of oncogenesis.
- Hereditary Retinoblastoma (germline mutations):

  In 40% of cases, retinoblastoma is caused by a germline mutation in the RB1 gene. These mutations are present in all cells of the body and can be passed from parent to child in autosomal dominant pattern. Individuals with a hereditary RB1 mutation have a higher risk of developing retinoblastoma in one or both eyes, as well as an increased risk of developing other types of cancers later in life.

- Non-hereditary Retinoblastoma (sporadic mutations):

  In the remaining 60% of cases, retinoblastoma is caused by a de novo mutation in the RB1 gene that occurs during early embryonic development. These mutations are not inherited from the parents and are present only in the cells that give rise to the retinoblastoma tumour. It typically affects only one eye.

Clinical manifestations

- Leukocoria - white or yellowish-white pupillary reflex in the affected eye, visible in certain lighting conditions, such as flash photography or dim light.
- Strabismus
- Decreased vision or visual impairment
- Eye pain or redness
- Poor fixation or following - inability to maintain steady eye contact
- Heterochromia - difference between the affected eye colour and the healthy eye
- Proptosis
- Secondary glaucoma
- Metastatic disease - retinoblastoma can metastasize to brain, bone marrow, or lymph nodes.
- Increased risk for pinealomas, osteosarcoma, soft tissue sarcomas and melanomas

Genetic Diagnosis

- Sequencing the RB1 gene using DNA obtained from peripheral blood or tumour tissue to identify pathogenic mutations that are associated with the condition. This also helps to differentiate somatic from germline mutation.

- Deletion/duplication analysis for RB1 gene can be done using Multiplex Ligation-dependent Probe Amplification (MLPA) or chromosomal microarray analysis (CMA).

Genetic counselling

- **Review of medical and family history**

  Gather detailed information about the affected individual's family history of Retinoblastoma or related conditions using a three-generational pedigree chart and consanguinity information. Details such as age of onset, laterality (unilateral or bilateral), vision loss, enucleation, secondary malignancies and treatment received and results of previous genetic testing should be noted. This assessment helps to determine the likelihood of an inherited genetic predisposition to retinoblastoma and guides recommendations for genetic testing and screening.

- **Discussion of Diagnosis**

  Counsellors must explain the role of the RB1 gene as a tumor suppressor and how its inactivation leads to uncontrolled cell division and tumorigenesis. The difference between heritable (germline) and non-heritable (somatic) forms must be clearly clarified. Emphasize that even if no family history is present, a germline mutation may still be the cause (due to de novo mutations). Symptoms such as leukocoria or strabismus should be linked to underlying tumor development.

- **Inheritance Pattern and Recurrence risk**

  Individuals with hereditary retinoblastoma have a 50% chance of transmitting the RB1 mutation to each of their children. The counsellor should discuss the likelihood of other family members being affected and provide information about genetic testing options for family members who may be at risk. Individuals with non-hereditary retinoblastoma do not have a family history of the condition, and their offspring are not at increased risk of inheriting the mutation. However, the counsellor should discuss the possibility of germline mosaicism and its implications.

- **Pre-test counselling**

  Explain the role of genetic testing in confirming a diagnosis of Retinoblastoma and determining the specific genetic mutation responsible for the condition. Discuss the benefits, limitations, and implications of genetic testing, including potential psychological and emotional considerations, and obtain informed consent before proceeding with testing.

- **Post-test counselling**

  Communicate the genetic test results to the individual or family, providing clear explanations and answering any questions or concerns that may arise. Interpret the test results in the context of the individual's medical and family history, explaining the implications of positive, negative, or inconclusive results. If pathogenic variant is found, at-risk family members should be offered genetic testing to identify those who carry the mutation and require early screening and management. For a negative result in unilateral, non-familial cases, reassure low familial risk, but recommend continued clinical vigilance.

- **Medical Management and Surveillance**

  Management includes enucleation, focal therapies, chemotherapy, and in select cases, radiation. Early detection allows for globe-sparing interventions. Lifelong surveillance is necessary for those with germline mutations due to the risk of second malignancies. Regular follow-ups with ophthalmologists, oncologists, and geneticists are essential for surveillance and support. All the first-degree relatives of the individual affected with hereditary retinoblastoma should have regular eye examination for early detection of malignancy.

- **Reproductive and Family Planning**

  If applicable, the counsellor should discuss reproductive options and family planning considerations for the affected individual and other family members, including prenatal testing, preimplantation genetic diagnosis (PGD), and gamete donation or adoption.

- **Psychosocial Support**

  Genetic counselling should include emotional support and guidance to help individuals and families cope with the challenges of living with Retinoblastoma. Address any concerns, fears, or psychosocial issues that the family may be experiencing and provide resources for additional support services, such as support groups or mental health counselling.

- **Follow-Up and Referrals**

  Schedule follow-up appointments as needed to monitor the individual's condition, provide ongoing support, and address any new questions or concerns that arise. Refer the family to other healthcare providers or specialists including ophthalmologists, oncologists, geneticists, and mental health professionals for multidisciplinary care.

- **Documentation**

  All genetic counselling sessions must be thoroughly documented, including family history, clinical findings, informed consent, test results, and the plan for management and follow-up. Genetic test reports should be stored securely with confidentiality.

References

1. Singh, L., Chinnaswamy, G., Meel, R., Radhakrishnan, V., Madan, R., Kulkarni, S., Sasi, A., Kaur, T., Dhaliwal, R. S., & Bakhshi, S. (2024). Epidemiology, Diagnosis and Genetics of Retinoblastoma: ICMR Consensus Guidelines. Indian journal of pediatrics, 91(11), 1147–1156.

2. Nag, A., & Khetan, V. (2024). Retinoblastoma - A comprehensive review, update and recent advances. Indian journal of ophthalmology, 72(6), 778–788.

3. Soliman, S. E., Racher, H., Zhang, C., MacDonald, H., & Gallie, B. L. (2017). Genetics and Molecular Diagnostics in Retinoblastoma--An Update. Asia-Pacific journal of ophthalmology (Philadelphia, Pa.), 6(2), 197–207.

4. DeBenedictis, M.J., Singh, A.D. (2019). Retinoblastoma: Genetic Counseling and Testing. In: Berry, J., Kim, J., Damato, B., Singh, A. (eds) Clinical Ophthalmic Oncology. Springer

OTHER DISORDERS

Alport Syndrome

Introduction

- Alport syndrome is a rare genetic disorder primarily affecting the kidneys, inner ear, and eyes.
- It is a progressive condition characterized by hematuria, proteinuria, sensorineural hearing loss, and ocular anomalies.
- Early diagnosis and intervention are crucial to slow the progression of kidney disease and manage extra-renal manifestations.

Genetic Etiology

- It results from mutations in genes encoding type IV collagen, a vital component of basement membranes in the kidney glomeruli, cochlea, and ocular structures.
- Mutations are observed in three genes, COL4A3, COL4A4, and COL4A5, which code for α3, α4, and α5 chains of type IV collagen.
- Alport syndrome can be inherited in three patterns.
- X-Linked Alport Syndrome (XLAS): This is the most common form, accounting for about 80-85% of cases. It is caused by mutations in the COL4A5 gene on the X chromosome. Males with XLAS are more severely affected, females show variable expressivity due to X-inactivation.

- Autosomal Recessive Alport Syndrome (ARAS): This form accounts for about 10-15% of cases and is caused by mutations in both copies of either the COL4A3 or COL4A4 genes. Both parents are obligate carriers.
- Autosomal Dominant Alport Syndrome (ADAS): Rare form, caused by heterozygous mutations in either COL4A3 or COL4A4 genes. It often results in a milder and more slowly progressive phenotype.

Clinical Manifestations

- Renal Symptoms: The hallmark of Alport syndrome is progressive kidney disease, often starting with hematuria and leading to proteinuria, eventually progressing to chronic kidney disease and end-stage renal disease (ESRD).
- Hearing Loss: Progressive bilateral sensorineural hearing loss typically develops in late childhood or early adolescence and often progresses with age.
- Eye Abnormalities: Include anterior lenticonus (bulging of the lens surface), which is unique to Alport syndrome, retinal flecks, recurrent corneal erosions, and posterior polymorphous dystrophy.
- Other Possible Features: Individuals may develop leiomyomatosis (smooth muscle tumors) in the esophagus, tracheobronchial tree or genital tract in some rare variants of the disorder.

Genetic Diagnosis

- Gene Sequencing: DNA sequencing of COL4A3, COL4A4, and COL4A5 helps in identifying specific pathogenic variants confirm the diagnosis. This is crucial for guiding prognosis, family planning, and cascade testing.
- MLPA or chromosomal microarray (CMA) is used to detect large deletions or duplications not easily picked up by sequencing, especially in COL4A5.

- Kidney Biopsy: Electron microscopy may reveal characteristic basement membrane changes (splitting and thickening), supporting the diagnosis.

Genetic Counselling

- **Review of Medical and Family History**

  Collect a detailed family history with three-generation pedigree and consanguinity information to understand inheritance patterns, potential de novo mutations, and recurrence risk. Use of a three-generation pedigree can help identify potential carriers and affected family members. Particular attention should be paid to unexplained kidney disease, hearing loss, or ocular abnormalities.

- **Discussion of Diagnosis**

  Explain Alport syndrome's nature, symptoms, progression, and potential complications, including kidney failure, hearing loss, and eye involvement. Discuss the specific inheritance pattern observed in the family.

- **Inheritance Pattern and Recurrence Risk**

  X-Linked Alport Syndrome (XLAS): Affected females have a 50% chance of passing the mutation to each child, regardless of sex. Sons who inherit the mutation will be affected, and daughters who inherit it will also be affected but with variable and milder symptoms. Affected males transmit the gene to all daughters, who become obligate carriers, but no male-to-male transmission. Outline the possibility of de novo mutations in the COL4A5 gene in approximately 15% of XLAS cases.

  Autosomal Recessive Alport Syndrome (ARAS): If both parents are carriers, each child has a 25% chance of being affected, a 50% chance of being a carrier, and a 25% chance of being unaffected.

  Autosomal Dominant Alport Syndrome (ADAS): If one parent is affected, each child has a 50% chance of inheriting the mutated gene and being affected. There is no carrier state for ADAS.

- **Pre-Test Counselling**

  Discuss the importance of genetic testing for confirming diagnosis, identifying inheritance patterns, and enabling cascade testing for at-risk family members. Clarify the limitations of genetic testing. Obtain informed consent for testing and address any potential psychological implications of knowing one's carrier or affected status. This includes discussing the impact of early knowledge on lifestyle, medical management, and reproductive planning.

- **Post-Test Counselling**

  Communicate the genetic test results, offer explanations, answer questions, and discuss its implications for diagnosis and prognosis of the condition. Discuss the benefits and process of cascade testing for at-risk relatives to identify asymptomatic individuals or carriers.

- **Medical Management and Surveillance**

  Regular monitoring of kidney function (urinalysis, blood tests) and blood pressure management, and lipid control are important. Patients may benefit from early intervention with angiotensin-converting enzyme (ACE) inhibitors to slow kidney disease progression. While cognitive function is usually preserved, sensorineural hearing loss can affect language development in children and should be screened early. Audiometry should be conducted periodically to monitor hearing loss, with recommendations for hearing aids or cochlear implants if necessary. Ophthalmology follow-up is advised, especially if eye abnormalities develop.

- **Reproductive and Family Planning**

  Options such as preimplantation genetic diagnosis (PGD) in conjunction with in vitro fertilization (IVF), and prenatal testing (chorionic villus sampling or amniocentesis) may be discussed with affected individuals or carrier couples to reduce transmission risk. Discuss the possibility of adoption or using donor gametes, if relevant.

- **Psychosocial Support**

  Provide essential emotional support and resources, addressing the significant impact of chronic kidney disease, hearing loss, and visual impairment on patients and families. Counselling should include the potential for guilt, anxiety, or stigma in carrier females and address coping strategies. Support groups and mental health resources may be suggested to aid coping and connect families with shared experiences.

- **Follow-Up and Referrals**

  Schedule regular follow-up appointments for ongoing support, periodic testing, and condition monitoring. Referrals to a multidisciplinary team including nephrologists, audiologists, ophthalmologists, and geneticists for comprehensive management and interdisciplinary care.

- **Documentation**

  Thorough documentation should include the family pedigree, relevant clinical findings, and genetic test reports with their interpretations. Informed consent forms, summaries of counselling discussions, and details of family planning or surveillance recommendations must also be recorded. All records must be securely stored and access limited to authorized personnel to ensure patient confidentiality.

References

1. Gregorio, V., Caparali, E. B., Shojaei, A., Ricardo, S., & Barua, M. (2023). Alport Syndrome: Clinical Spectrum and Therapeutic Advances. Kidney medicine, 5(5), 100631.
2. Nozu, K., Yamamura, T., & Horinouchi, T. (2001). Alport Syndrome. In M. P. Adam (Eds.) et. al. (2022). Guidelines for Genetic Testing and Management of Alport Syndrome. Clinical journal of the American Society of Nephrology : CJASN, 17(1), 143–154.

3. Kashtan C. E. (2021). Alport Syndrome: Achieving Early Diagnosis and Treatment. American journal of kidney diseases : the official journal of the National Kidney Foundation, 77(2), 272–279.

4. Savige J, Ariani F, Mari F, et al. Expert guidelines for the genetic diagnosis of Alport syndrome. Pediatr Nephrol. 2019;34(7):1175-1189.

5. Fernandez-Rosado, F., Campos, A., Alvarez-Cubero, M. J., Ruiz, A., & Entrala-Bernal, C. (2015). Improved genetic counseling in Alport syndrome by new variants of COL4A5 gene. Nephrology (Carlton, Vic.), 20(7), 502–505.

Non-Syndromic Hearing Loss

Introduction

- Non-syndromic hearing loss (NSHL) refers to isolated sensorineural hearing impairment that occurs without other associated clinical abnormalities or dysmorphic features
- NSHL accounts for approximately 70% of genetic hearing loss cases.
- It can be congenital or late-onset, stable or progressive, and may vary in severity from mild to profound.
- It may present unilaterally or bilaterally, though bilateral involvement is more common.
- Genetic causes are highly heterogeneous, involving over 150 identified genes.

Genetic Etiology

- Over 150 genes have been implicated in NSHL; the most common mutations occur in the *GJB2* gene (connexin 26) and GJB6.
- Autosomal recessive NSHL (ARNSHL) accounts for about 80% of inherited NSHL, with *GJB2*, *SLC26A4*, and *OTOF* being common genes.
- Autosomal dominant NSHL (ADNSHL) represents about 15-20% of inherited NSHL and is often postlingual and progressive. Common ADNSHL genes include KCNQ4, MYO6, and WFS1.

- X-linked and mitochondrial forms are rare but significant, especially for syndromic differentials.
- Environmental factors, like perinatal infections and ototoxic drugs, must be excluded before considering a genetic etiology.

Clinical Manifestation

- Congenital or early-onset bilateral sensorineural hearing loss.
- Absence of dysmorphic features or systemic manifestations.
- Hearing loss may be stable or progressive, and of variable severity.
- Family history may reveal consanguinity or affected relatives with isolated hearing loss.
- Language development may be delayed in undiagnosed cases.

Genetic Diagnosis

- Newborn hearing screening: Otoacoustic emissions (OAE) or auditory brainstem response (ABR) tests.
- GJB2 gene sequencing: First-tier test in many populations due to high mutation prevalence.
- Multigene panels using next-generation sequencing (NGS): Useful when *GJB2* is negative.
- Copy number variation (CNV) analysis and deletion/duplication testing: Detect large deletions (e.g., del(GJB6-D13S1830), which can occur in trans to a GJB2 mutation, causing ARNSHL).
- Mitochondrial DNA analysis: Recommended for maternally inherited hearing loss or aminoglycoside-induced ototoxicity.
- SLC26A4 testing and temporal bone imaging: Indicated when enlarged vestibular aqueduct is present.

Genetic Counselling

- **Review of Medical and Family History**

  A thorough review should include a three-generation pedigree with specific attention to consanguinity, history of childhood or adult-onset hearing loss, exposure to ototoxic drugs, maternal infections during pregnancy (e.g., CMV, Rubella), and perinatal complications. Inquire about other affected family members and syndromic features (e.g., vision loss, kidney disease, cardiac issues, thyroid dysfunction, balance problems) to rule out associated conditions that would indicate a syndromic form of hearing loss.

- **Discussion of Diagnosis**

  Explain that non-syndromic hearing loss is genetically heterogeneous and commonly inherited in an autosomal recessive pattern. Emphasize that the absence of other symptoms defines NSHL and differentiates it from syndromic forms. If testing identifies a pathogenic variant, link the genotype with the phenotype and explain implications for hearing, prognosis.

- **Inheritance Pattern**

  Discuss the most likely inheritance based on clinical and molecular findings. ARNSHL is the most common, with a 25% recurrence risk if both parents are carriers. ADNSHL carries a 50% risk of transmission to each child. X-linked and mitochondrial inheritance patterns are rare but should be considered when suggested by pedigree analysis or maternal inheritance. Explain the potential for de novo mutations in ADNSHL, which would mean a very low recurrence risk for parents but 50% for the affected individual's offspring.

- **Pre-test Counselling**

  Pre-test counselling should cover the benefits, limitations, and implications of genetic testing. Informed consent must be obtained, especially if testing may reveal incidental findings or reproductive implications. Families should understand that a negative result does not rule out a genetic cause due to current testing limitations.

- **Post-test Counselling**

  Results must be interpreted in clinical context. For pathogenic variants, discuss recurrence risks and implications for family screening. Offer cascade testing to at-risk relatives. Inconclusive results (Variants of Uncertain Significance - VUS) should be explained with options for future reanalysis or family segregation studies to aid interpretation. Negative results may require re-evaluation if phenotype evolves or if new genes or technologies emerge.

- **Medical Management and Surveillance**

  Management involves timely audiologic interventions such as hearing aids, cochlear implants, or sign language training. Early intervention significantly improves language outcomes. Monitor for progression and comorbidities, even if the hearing loss is initially stable. Surveillance should be according to the specific genetic cause when known.

- **Reproductive and Family Planning**

  Inform parents of recurrence risks and reproductive options, including carrier screening, preimplantation genetic diagnosis (PGD), and prenatal testing for confirmed familial variants. Discuss options such as donor gametes and adoption if both partners are carriers of a recessive condition and desire to avoid the recurrence risk.

- **Psychosocial Support**

  Hearing loss can affect communication, learning, and social development. Offer referrals to local and regional support groups, such as those for hearing-impaired children and families. Encourage connecting with community networks and peer mentors to reduce isolation and enhance coping strategies.

- **Follow-Up and Referrals**

  Follow-up should include ongoing coordination with audiologists, ENT specialists, pediatricians, and speech/language therapists. Referral to a clinical geneticist is recommended for complex cases or when extended family screening is required.

- **Documentation**

  Ensure accurate documentation of the family pedigree, test results, counselling discussion, and consent forms. Maintain secure records with appropriate privacy safeguards. All recommendations and referrals should be recorded, and summary reports shared with relevant clinicians with appropriate consent.

References

1. Shearer AE, Hildebrand MS, Smith RJH. Hereditary Hearing Loss and Deafness Overview. *GeneReviews*. Updated 2023.
2. Vona, B., Nanda, I., Hofrichter, M. A., Shehata-Dieler, W., & Haaf, T. (2015). Non-syndromic hearing loss gene identification: A brief history and glimpse into the future. Molecular and cellular probes, 29(5), 260–270.
3. Funamura J. L. (2017). Evaluation and management of nonsyndromic congenital hearing loss. Current opinion in otolaryngology & head and neck surgery, 25(5), 385–389.
4. Gooch, C., Rudy, N., Smith, R. J., & Robin, N. H. (2021). Genetic testing hearing loss: The challenge of non syndromic mimics. International journal of pediatric otorhinolaryngology, 150, 110872.

Primary Amenorrhea

Introduction

- Primary amenorrhea is defined as the absence of menstruation by age 15 or 3 years after thelarche.
- It is a clinical sign rather than a diagnosis, with diverse etiologies including genetic, anatomical, hormonal, and systemic causes.
- Genetic counselling is crucial, especially in cases with chromosomal, monogenic, or complex etiologies, as it impacts diagnosis, prognosis, and reproductive planning.

Genetic Etiology

- Turner syndrome (45,X) and its variants (e.g., 45,X/46,XX mosaicism) are common chromosomal causes.
- Androgen insensitivity syndrome (AIS) results from mutations in the AR gene on the X chromosome.
- 46,XY gonadal dysgenesis (Swyer syndrome) may involve mutations in SRY or other sex-determining genes, resulting in streak gonads and lack of male sex development.
- Congenital anomalies like Müllerian agenesis (MRKH syndrome) may have a familial basis but are often sporadic.
- Other gene mutations associated include CYP17A1, NR5A1, and GALT (in galactosemia-related cases).

Clinical Manifestation

- Absence of menstruation by expected age.
- Normal or delayed secondary sexual development depending on the underlying cause.
- Possible short stature, webbed neck (Turner syndrome), or tall stature with sparse pubic hair (AIS).
- Normal external genitalia in most cases; internal genitalia may be absent or dysgenetic.
- May present with cyclic abdominal pain if outflow tract obstruction exists.

Genetic Diagnosis

- Karyotyping: Essential for evaluating chromosomal abnormalities such as Turner syndrome (45,X) or 46,XY disorders of sex development.
- FISH or chromosomal microarray: To identify mosaicism or sub-microscopic deletions.
- Gene sequencing: For suspected monogenic causes (e.g., AR, SRY, NR5A1, CYP17A1).
- Pelvic ultrasound or MRI: To assess the presence of uterus and ovaries.
- Hormonal profile: FSH, LH, estrogen, prolactin, AMH, TSH to guide towards central (hypothalamic/pituitary) or peripheral causes (ovarian/anatomical).

Genetic Counselling

- **Review of Medical and Family History**

  A thorough clinical history and three-generation pedigree should be obtained, focusing on age at menarche in family members, consanguinity, history of delayed puberty, infertility, or other reproductive anomalies. Growth patterns, developmental milestones, and history of neonatal issues should also be documented.

- **Discussion of Diagnosis**

  The counsellor should correlate clinical findings (e.g., short stature, lack of pubertal signs) with diagnostic results. Explain the implications of karyotype findings (e.g., Turner syndrome, 46,XY DSD), hormone profiles, and gene test outcomes. Emphasize that primary amenorrhea is a symptom with multiple genetic and non-genetic causes. Acknowledge the emotional impact of a diagnosis that may affect fertility or gender identity.

- **Inheritance Pattern and Recurrence Risk**

  Inheritance varies by etiology: Turner syndrome is usually sporadic; AIS is X-linked recessive; SRY-related disorders are often de novo but can rarely be familial; CYP17A1 and NR5A1 mutations may follow autosomal recessive or dominant patterns. Mosaicism adds complexity to inheritance and phenotype variability, and can influence recurrence risk for parents.

- **Pre-test Counselling**

  Before genetic testing, explain the purpose of tests such as karyotyping, gene panels, and hormonal assessments. Informed consent must be obtained, especially when identifying disorders of sex development. Potential psychological impact of findings must be anticipated and addressed sensitively.

- **Post-test Counselling**

  Communicate the results clearly, explaining their clinical relevance and implications for health, fertility, and recurrence risks. If a genetic diagnosis is made, cascade testing for at-risk relatives may be advised. Provide anticipatory guidance on next steps for medical or surgical management.

- **Medical Management and Surveillance**

  Management is condition-specific and requires a multidisciplinary care. Medical therapy may include hormone replacement therapy (estrogen/progesterone) for pubertal induction and maintenance of secondary sexual characteristics in cases of gonadal dysgenesis or hypogonadotropic hypogonadism. Gonadectomy is recommended in 46,XY DSD with streak gonads or undescended testes due to malignancy risk. Surgical correction may be necessary for outflow tract obstructions. Monitor for associated complications such as osteoporosis, cardiovascular issues, renal anomalies, and gonadal tumors.

- **Reproductive and Family Planning**

  Discuss fertility potential based on diagnosis: individuals with primary ovarian insufficiency will typically require oocyte donation with IVF. Individuals with certain forms of 46,XY DSD may have some sperm production but often require assisted reproduction. For individuals with Müllerian agenesis, surrogacy may be an option. PGD and prenatal testing may be applicable for inherited forms or when a specific familial genetic risk is identified. Counselling should be customised to respect cultural values, psychosocial readiness, and the individual's long-term reproductive goals.

- **Psychosocial Support**

  Address emotional and psychological implications, particularly regarding gender identity, body image, and infertility. Referral to psychologists specializing in DSD or reproductive health, and support groups is strongly recommended. Long-term psychosocial support may be required for coping and adjustment throughout different life stages.

- **Follow-Up and Referrals**

  Coordinate ongoing follow-up with endocrinologists, gynecologists, geneticists, and mental health professionals. Multidisciplinary care ensures optimal management of medical, reproductive, and psychosocial aspects. Annual reviews are essential for therapy adherence, monitoring complications, and addressing evolving needs.

- **Documentation**

  Maintain comprehensive records including clinical findings, pedigree, informed consent, test results, and counselling notes. Ensure all documentation is securely stored with strict confidentiality, and summary reports are shared with relevant healthcare providers with appropriate consent.

References

1. Yatsenko, S. A., Witchel, S. F., & Gordon, C. M. (2024). Primary Amenorrhea and Premature Ovarian Insufficiency. Endocrinology and metabolism clinics of North America, 53(2), 293–305.
2. Marsh, C. A., & Grimstad, F. W. (2014). Primary amenorrhea: diagnosis and management. Obstetrical & gynecological survey, 69(10), 603–612.
3. Herlin, M. K., Petersen, M. B., & Brännström, M. (2020). Mayer-Rokitansky-Küster-Hauser (MRKH) syndrome: a comprehensive update. Orphanet journal of rare diseases, 15(1), 214.
4. Gaspari L, Paris F, Kalfa N, Sultan C. Primary Amenorrhea in Adolescents: Approach to Diagnosis and Management. *Endocrines*. 2023; 4(3):536-547.

www.ingramcontent.com/pod-product-compliance
Ingram Content Group UK Ltd.
Pitfield, Milton Keynes, MK11 3LW, UK
UKHW022025190726
13853UKWH00005B/2122

9 798899 847813